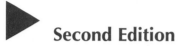

Second Edition

Childhood Motor
Speech Disability

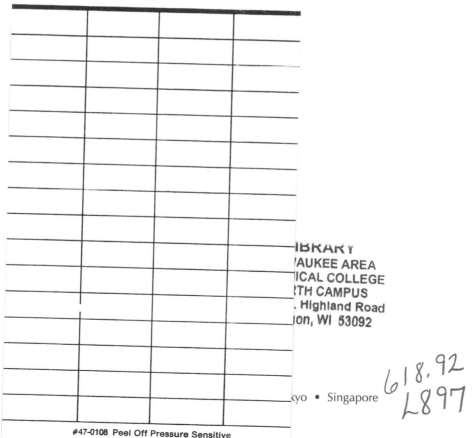

DATE DUE

#47-0108 Peel Off Pressure Sensitive

kyo • Singapore

To a superb teacher of speech-language pathology,
Harold Westlake, Ph.D., and the memory of a brilliant,
fascinating, and caring father, Abraham I. Love, M.D.

Executive Editor: Stephen D. Dragin
Vice President, Editor-in-Chief: Paul A. Smith
Editorial Assistant: Bridget McSweeney
Senior Marketing Manager: Brad Parkins
Production Editor: Christopher H. Rawlings
Editorial-Production Service: Omegatype Typography, Inc.
Composition and Prepress Buyer: Linda Cox
Manufacturing Buyer: David Repetto
Cover Administrator: Jenny Hart
Electronic Composition: Omegatype Typography, Inc.

Library of Congress Cataloging-in-Publication Data

Love, Russell J.
    Childhood motor speech disability / Russell J. Love. — 2nd ed.
        p.   cm.
    Includes bibliographical references and index.
    ISBN 0-205-29781-1 (pbk.)
    1. Speech disorders in children.   2. Cerebral palsied children.
I. Title.
    [DNLM: 1. Dysarthria—Child.   2. Language Development Disorders—
physiopathology.   3. Motor Skills—physiology.   4. Speech
Disorders—Child.   WL 340 L897c 2000]
RJ496.S7L68   2000
618.92'855—dc21
DNLM/DLC
for Library of Congress   99-16113
                                                                        CIP

Printed in the United States of America
10 9 8 7 6 5 4 3 2   04   03   02   01   00

Contents

Preface

The goal of this edition is to present a balanced but critical view of the significant literature in childhood motor speech disorders (CMSD) that has appeared since 1992. In most cases, this new and recent material demands a new set of revised and refined interpretations of earlier thought about CMSD. In a few cases, a healthy skepticism is aroused about the validity of some reported research results. A review of the research in certain areas of CMSD raises questions about the current direction our research programs in motor speech disorders are taking. We find obvious strengths, and also glaring weaknesses, in our overall research planning in this field.

One minor but important change in Chapter 1 is an attempt to underline the need for a consistent and clearer classification of the childhood dysarthrias. I believe the classification system used in this book is the most acceptable available because it encompasses the best of the older classifications.

There is essentially no change in the neurology of motor systems (Chapter 2) and the clinical description of the dysarthrias of cerebral palsy (Chapter 3). The lower motor neuron dysarthrias (Chapter 4) remain unchanged by the passage of time since the first edition.

Our discussion of the use of surgery to control severe and chronic drooling in highly selective cases of cerebral palsy (Chapter 7) aroused more comment among physicians and speech-language pathologists than I had expected. Repositioning of the parotid glands that excrete saliva, it was said, was a hazard to good oral hygiene. Before use of surgery, most physicians recommended a trial of drug treatment.[1]

If the drug is not completely effective, surgery may be considered. Ronald Swang, D.D.S., has brought his wide experience and knowledge to the issues involved in drooling surgery. His thoughtful opinions offer sensible solutions to arguments, pro and con, about repositioning the parotid glands. I am indebted to Dr. Swang for his help with this many-faceted problem.

---

[1]K. M. Yorkston, D. R. Beukelman, and E. A. Strand report the use of glycopyrolate as a current drug that is helpful in the treatment of chronic drooling (*Management of Motor Speech Disorders in Children and Adults*, 2nd ed., Austin, TX: Pro-ed, 1999, p. 42).

To me, the topic of developmental verbal dyspraxia (DVD) is the most controversial one in the whole area of child motor speech disorders (Chapter 5). It has received an inordinate amount of attention lately in the speech-language pathology literature, considering that it is known as a low-frequency communication disorder among the significantly greater number of children with unexplained phonologic delay to which it is often compared. Nevertheless, DVD is occupying the research efforts of several investigators who see it as a subset of early idiopathic phonologic delay. I think the reader will find that the many and varied arguments about this uncommon phonologic disorder will add up to a "good read" among the more prosaic discussions seen in the pediatric literature on other communication disorders.

Since its advent, the personal computer has appealed to individuals working with severe disabilities. It seemed to be a ready technological panacea for dealing with individuals who were speechless or near-speechless. The computer appeared ideal for cases that would benefit from augmentative or alternative communication approaches. Therefore, in the past few years considerable research time has been expended to determine the potential use of the computer with such severely disabled individuals. Some of this recent research is reviewed in Chapter 7, and the issues involved in using computers appear to be very complex. The research has established that there are numerous variables, some yet unknown, involved in achieving successful computer competence in communication. It seems to be a model of the type of investigation that must be completed to alter radically the communication skills of the severely communicatively impaired for the better.

However, the promise of this type of research excellence is not apparent in the work being reported in the area of therapy approaches for developmental verbal apraxia. Experimental replication of so-called successful therapy approaches is not being reported at all, so we are unable to verify the most promising management techniques for DVD from among the wide array of suggested approaches. In other words, we are without a scientific basis for our clinical practices. Hopefully I will be able to report progress in this area in a third edition. Our field sorely needs it, as do our child clients.

I am deeply indebted to several people for the successful completion of this book. My longtime friend and collaborator Wanda G. Webb, Ph.D., Vanderbilt University, performed needed library research and reviewed the manuscript for me. My devoted wife, Barbara, did the necessary cutting and pasting of the manuscript as well as the word processing. Two departmental secretaries, Judy Warren and Kathy Rhody, went beyond the call of duty, allowing me to offer a presentable manuscript to my affable and encouraging editor, Stephen Dragin. Finally, I wish to acknowledge Fred H. Bess, Ph.D., chairman of my university department. He has been extremely supportive of my work during "the emeritus years" of my career.

► 1

The Nature of Childhood Motor Speech Disability

The muscles of speech are commonly involved, varying in degree from inability to utter correctly a particular letter to the entire loss of articulating power. Sometimes articulation is only slow and difficult . . .
—WILLIAM JOHN LITTLE, 1861

INTRODUCTION: CHILDHOOD DYSARTHRIA
VERSUS DEVELOPMENTAL VERBAL DYSPRAXIA

Motor speech disability refers to speech impairment caused by a lesion or dysfunction of motor control centers in either the peripheral or central nervous systems or in a combination of both systems. The result is an inability to regulate the movements of the speech musculature. In modern clinical usage, the term *motor speech disability* encompasses two broad categories: (1) dysarthria and (2) apraxia of speech. These two terms were introduced into clinical neurology early in its history and are associated with Charcot (1877) and Leipmann (1908), respectively. Although these terms have widely been used to designate major speech disorders in adults in both neurology and speech-language pathology, there is incomplete agreement as to what nomenclature should be used to distinguish motor speech disability in children. In this book, the terms *childhood dysarthria* and *developmental verbal dyspraxia* will be employed to designate the subcategories of childhood motor speech disability. The reasons for choosing these terms will become apparent from discussions in later sections of this chapter.

Distinguishing between the two major childhood speech disabilities is sometimes very difficult, because in both instances the defining symptom—deviant speech—is caused by somewhat similar awkward movements of the speech muscles. In some cases, this defining symptom is part of a larger clinical picture that points to the appropriate diagnosis. For example, the stormy birth history, the delayed motor development, the feeding difficulties, and the generalized paralysis or abnormal movements of the cerebral-palsied child make it highly likely that the awkward speech movements are the basis of a dysarthria rather than of a verbal dyspraxia. In contrast, normal birth and developmental histories, awkward speech movements with no paralysis or weakness of the oral muscles, and equivocal signs of neurologic impairment are highly suggestive of a diagnosis of developmental verbal dyspraxia in a child.

To clarify the differences between what at first may appear to be only variations of the same speech disorder, consider the case histories of two 7-year-old children referred to a speech-language pathologist for evaluation.

Case 1: *Childhood Dysarthria*

Julie, now 7 years, 5 months of age, has been brought by her parents for speech assessment as part of a team evaluation at the cerebral palsy clinic of a large university medical center. The purpose of the team evaluation is to make recommendations for school placement. Julie has been followed at the cerebral palsy clinic since the age of 2 years, 2 months. Past medical history reveals cerebral hypoxia at birth from a prolapsed umbilical cord. The delivery was a breech presentation; it was immediately followed by seizure activity and resuscitation for a 20-minute period. Medication for seizure control was administered for six months with no further convulsive incidents.

Developmental milestones were reached slowly. Julie sat alone at 13 months, crawled at 24 months, and reportedly said her first word approximation at 10 months. At the first evaluation, her parents reported no major feeding problems in early infancy, but the speech pathology notes in the patient's chart indicate obvious motor involvement of the oral musculature along with excessive drooling. Good anterior-posterior tongue movement was observed with adequate protrusion and retraction of the tongue. Minimal lateralization and elevation of the tongue tip were present. Phonation was initiated with difficulty and was not easily sustained. Articulation was distorted with bilabial and alveolar phonemes predominating in the speech pattern.

Receptive and expressive language at 20 months was reported within normal range. Speech reception thresholds in a sound field were normal, and impedance audiometry demonstrated normal pressure compliance. Acoustic reflexes were absent bilaterally, and it was recommended that pure tone audiometry be completed as soon as conditioning for the task could be accomplished. The *Bayley Scales of Infant Development* (Bayley, 1969) suggested overall performance at the 22-months level with a chronological age of 26 months, but Julie passed receptive language items at her age level. Results of the *Revised Stanford-Binet Intelligence Scale (Form L-M)* (Terman & Merrill, 1973) indicated that Julie completed form discrimination and body-part identification at the 2½-year level. Her overall mental functioning was judged within normal limits.

Neurologic evaluation revealed that the cranial nerves were grossly intact. Muscle tone was increased in all extremities, particularly in the legs. Deep tendon reflexes were brisk, and the Babinski sign was ambiguous. Tight heel cords were present bilaterally. The examining pediatric neurologist diagnosed a moderate-to-severe spasticity with a severe dysarthria.

Now at 7 years, Julie can walk by herself indoors with a wide-based gait and occasional moments of poor balance. During ambulation, accessory movement is present in the extremities. Outdoors, Julie uses crutches. She has had orthopedic surgery for bilateral transfer of hip adductors as well as bilateral heel-cord lengthening. Neurologic examination now reveals a diffuse hypertonicity with increased tendon reflexes in the range of 2+ to 3+ without deformity or contractures. Julie picks up small objects with some intention tremor and hand posturing. Some athetotic features of involuntary movement are present.

The psychologist notes that Julie is a cheerful, cooperative child who appears to comprehend all that is said to her. Her language, while understood in context, is more difficult to understand out of context; her mother was present during psychological testing to interpret some of the verbal responses. Her score on the verbal subtest of the *Wechsler Intelligence Scale for Children— Revised* (Wechsler, 1974) was 109, within normal limits.

Julie received speech and language training in a parent-infant language development program from the age of 2 years, 9 months until she was 3 years old. She then entered a local Easter Seal Society nursery school program and simultaneously received language stimulation, articulation therapy, and oral exercise training at a large community hearing and speech center. Later, her speech therapy at the center emphasized articulation improvement in phrases, sentences, and conversational attempts.

Speech evaluation today reveals that Julie is clearly a dysarthric speaker with reduced intelligibility. A breathing problem affects speech phrasing frequently. Julie can utter four to five syllables per breath, often relying on residual air to complete her utterances. A harsh voice quality is predominant and inconsistent hypernasality is occasionally heard. Excessive loudness and poor pitch control with frequent pitch breaks are present. The pitch is monotonous, and the speaking rate is slow.

Articulatory testing shows 59% of her phonemes in single words are in error. Substitutions and omissions of phonemes are the most common errors. Stimulability for later developing phonemes is poor.

Precise tongue-tip elevation is inconsistent, and there are slow and limited movements of the articulators. Athetotic movements of the tongue are seen, and facial grimaces are present. Syllable diadochokinetic rates are approximately 50% poorer than expectation for age. The speech diagnosis is a severe mixed spastic-athetotic dysarthria of cerebral palsy.

Recommendations include continued speech therapy, stressing articulation improvement and breath-control drills for improved speech phrasing. Therapy in the school setting as well as at a local speech and hearing center is planned. In addition, placement in an ungraded primary special education program at a parochial academy is recommended. Mainstreaming into a regular classroom at the academy is urged as soon as it is appropriate. Special supportive help for the general motor involvement is outlined for the school setting.

Case 2: *Developmental Verbal Dyspraxia*

Greg, 7 years, 9 months of age, has been tentatively diagnosed as exhibiting developmental verbal dyspraxia, superseding a previous diagnosis in the public schools of functional articulation disorder with learning disabilities. He is seen at this evaluation to confirm or deny that tentative diagnosis. Articulation age on the *Fisher-Logemann Test of Articulation Competence* (Fisher & Logemann, 1971) falls between 4 and 5 years. Phoneme errors analyzed in terms of the place of articulation are more frequent in the lingual-dental, lingual-alveolar, and lingual-palatal categories in both words and sentences. The manner of articulation analysis indicates that affricatives, glides, and fricatives, in that order, are most frequently misarticulated. The analysis points to particular difficulty in lingual motor control. In addition, prosodic disturbances are characterized by a slow rate and uneven stress. Overall speech intelligibility is poor.

Oral examination reveals that Greg is now able, on command, to produce voluntary movements of the articulators, a skill lacking in previous examinations. The strength, accuracy, and range of articulator movement are judged as fair in isolated movements. He appears to present a resolving oral dyspraxia but still retains elements of a possible verbal dyspraxia. Repetitive movements of the tongue are imprecise in syllable production and deteriorate with increased speech. Diadochokinetic rates for speech are reduced. In three trials of 5 seconds each, Greg produces the sequence /pʌ,tʌ,kʌ/ with three (100% correct), four (50% correct), and five (20% correct) repetitions. This reduced articulation programming ability is highly suggestive of a possible developmental verbal dyspraxia.

To rule out a childhood dysarthria, the oral muscles were examined for hypotonus and hypertonus. Signs of muscle-tone disturbance were absent. Involuntary and uncoordinated movements of the oral musculature, suggesting cerebellar or basal ganglia disorder, were not observed. The gag and jaw reflexes were normal. No vocal deviations characteristic of the dysarthrias were heard. The attending physician reports no "soft" neurologic signs that suggest minimal cerebral dysfunction. In his pediatric examination, he found no neurologic disturbances in the motor system.

Greg was first seen at a hearing and speech center at the age of 2 years, 5 months. Family history was essentially negative except that the father reported that he, himself, was slow to talk. Greg's birth history was normal. The prenatal, perinatal, and postnatal courses were without incident. Greg sat at 6 months, crawled at 10 months, and walked at 12 months. His medical history was unremarkable except for bouts of serous otitis media and a tight lingual frenulum.

Greg had approximately a dozen word approximations at this first evaluation. He communicated primarily with hand gestures and unintelligible jargon.

Oral examination indicated he had difficulty performing oral movements on command. During testing he was able to protrude and retract the tongue but had specific difficulty in elevating the tongue tip and in lateralizing it. Drooling was intermittently present. Oral movements appeared impaired in both speech and nonspeech activities. A mild ankyloglossia (tongue-tie) was relieved by surgery approximately one year after the initial speech evaluation; however, the expected recovery and achievement of normal motor patterns for speech did not occur, and inaccurate groping movements of the speech articulators persisted to the present evaluation, some four and a half years later.

Test results at the present evaluation from the *Goldman-Fristoe-Woodcock Auditory Skills Battery* (1974) indicate difficulty in selective attention (figure-background), sound-syllable skills, including sound analysis, sound blending, reading, and spelling. Further, specific language deficits in word processing and sentence structure, understanding linguistic concepts, producing names on confrontation, and making word associations are demonstrated on Wiig and Semmel's *Clinical Evaluation of Language Functions* (1980).

Greg was enrolled in a parent-infant language development program at 3 years of age and received speech therapy in the public schools as well as private articulation therapy during the summers until the current evaluation. He reportedly performed adequately in kindergarten and first grade but required considerable tutoring in his school work. His grades were described as average. His school performance prior to this evaluation prompted psychoeducational assessment with the following tests: *Wechsler Intelligence Scale for Children-Revised* (Wechsler, 1974), *California Achievement Test* (Tiegs & Clark, 1957), *Wide Range Achievement Test* (Jastak, 1965), and *The Bender Gestalt Test for Young Children* (Koppitz, 1964). Greg's performance was characterized by low average functioning with no discrepancy between ability and achievement. The speech reevaluation today confirms the earlier diagnosis of suspected developmental verbal dyspraxia.

Julie and Greg present very different birth histories, courses of development, educational careers, and clinical neuropathologic pictures. These differences act as strong supporting evidence for a differential diagnosis of either dysarthria or verbal dyspraxia. However, it should be noted that if the supporting evidence from case histories and motor examination of the extremities is discounted, the two companion disorders may appear almost identical on the basis of speech and oral performance alone. In fact, Stark (1985) points out that it remains difficult even in adults to separate dysarthria and verbal dyspraxia, but that in children, in whom the neural mechanisms are still under development, the distinction often may be impossible. This diagnostic dilemma, however, can be resolved to a certain extent by defining the disorders clearly and by understanding the major characteristic of each motor speech disability.

DEFINITION OF TERMS

Childhood Dysarthria

Childhood dysarthria is a neurogenic speech impairment caused by dysfunction of the motor control centers of the immature central and/or peripheral nervous systems and marked by disturbances of strength, speed, steadiness, coordination, precision, tone, and range of movement in the speech musculature. The term *dysarthria* typically designates a partial disturbance of speech because of motor involvement, while *anarthria* denotes complete lack of speech because of severe motor involvement.

The abnormal movements in speech are usually described clinically in a neurologic context with the following adjectives: weak or slow (as in paralysis), unsteady (as in tremor), uncoordinated (as in dysmetria or dyssynergia), hypotonic or hypertonic (as in decreased or increased muscle tone), and limited range of movement. Speech-language pathologists are often confused by the fact that these are subjective terms derived from descriptions of motor disturbances of the limbs and trunk that have a long history in neurologic medicine but may not always apply to disturbances of oral muscles. In fact, Abbs, Hunker, and Barlow (1983) have shown that there are a number of significant differences in physiologic and neurophysiologic control for the subsystems that govern speech movements and limb movements. Descriptive terminology employed for the disturbances in the limbs therefore may not always be appropriate for oral motor deviations.

Further, motor speech impairment is not always completely predictable on the basis of limb impairment in dysarthric individuals. Despite these limitations, the current terminology for motor disturbances is widely accepted in clinical neurology, and some terms still retain a certain communicative utility for designating the salient features of motor deviations in the oral muscles. Until a new set of operational terms is defined to describe oral motor deviations, it is likely the current terminology that is so well entrenched in neurology can be adapted by the speech-language pathologist to describe abnormal speech motor patterns.

The term *childhood dysarthria* itself actually implies a class of disorders, not a single disorder with an invariant set of speech signs and symptoms. Dysarthric patterns in children may vary with their age of onset, the underlying primary disease or neurologic condition, the site of lesion, and the number and severity of the speech subsystems involved in a given dysarthria.

Childhood dysarthria must be differentiated from other conditions that produce developmental communication disorders. In addition to being differentiated from verbal dyspraxia, dysarthria in its milder forms must be diagnostically differentiated from a developmental phonologic impairment of nonorganic origin, a so-called functional articulation disorder. Generally, a dysarthria is marked by unequivocal motor involvement of the speech musculature, a positive neurologic history, and demonstrable neurologic signs independent of motor involvement of the speech systems, all of which tend to support a diagnosis of organicity of the speech problem. If, however, the dysarthria is extremely mild and the child presents an inconclusive history of cerebral dysfunction, the speech pattern easily may be confused with one of developmental phonologic impairment (Stark, 1985).

In addition, childhood dysarthria must be separated from language delay or disorder. In many cases of dysarthria, the neurologic impairment that produces the motor speech disability is also responsible for lowered intelligence. A concomitant language delay will therefore exist.

Beyond developmental language delay, the question of whether certain specific language deficits coexist in childhood dysarthric populations has been frequently raised (Bishop, 1988; Flower, Viebweg, & Ruzicka, 1966; Love, 1964; Myers, 1965). Another unanswered question is whether either dysarthria or anarthria has a major effect on the ability to understand and use verbal processing in mental operations (Bishop, Brown, & Robson, 1990).

Developmental Verbal Dyspraxia

Developmental verbal dyspraxia (DVD), also known as **developmental apraxia of speech** (DAS), is an impaired ability of the child, in the absence of obvious muscular disturbance of the speech mechanism, to execute voluntarily the expected motor gestures and programming of gestures needed for the articulation of speech. A striking feature of DVD or DAS is the child's inability to produce an appropriate motor gesture for speech but yet demonstrate the same motor gesture in a more automatic nonverbal act. The child, for instance, may be unable to elevate the tongue tip to the gum ridge for a lingual-alveolar phoneme but during the act of eating may easily raise the tongue to the gum ridge to lick off a bit of food adhering to it. This suggests that the inability to produce tongue-tip action for speech units is not the same as the motor involvement observed in childhood dysarthria wherein movements for speech and mastication are similarly involved. In brief, the disability in developmental verbal dyspraxia is one of voluntary motor programming and sequencing of speech rather than one of motor force and control in both speech and nonspeech acts, as is the case in childhood dysarthria.

Developmental Oral Apraxia

On occasion, the term *developmental oral apraxia* has been used synonymously for DVD and DAS, but most communication specialists reserve it for a related but distinctly different disorder of praxis of the oral facial muscles in children. Specifically, **developmental oral apraxia** is an inability to perform voluntary movements of the muscles of the pharynx, tongue, cheeks, and lips, although automatic movements of these muscles may be preserved. In other words, it is an apraxia of nonspeech acts.

Neurologists generally believe that this disorder, often called buccofacial apraxia in adults, is the primary cause for a speech dyspraxia in Broca's aphasia (Hier, Gorelick, & Shindler, 1987); however, there is evidence that some adults have apraxic speech without bucco-facial apraxia (DeRenzi, Pieczuro, & Vignolo, 1966; Wertz, La Pointe, & Rosenbek, 1984). It is unclear whether similar relationships hold true in children suspected of DVD. Aram and Nation (1982) are of the opinion that these two conditions may either be independent or coexist with each other in children.

Theoretical Distinctions

Theoretical distinctions for differentiating child dysarthria and DVD can be derived from neurologic models of language and speech production in adults (Buckingham, 1981; Darley, Aronson, & Brown, 1975), as well as from newer psycholinguistic models of speech production and speech motor control in the adult (Levett, 1989). These theoretical distinctions can be useful in understanding the two disorders. Classical neurology places verbal and oral dyspraxic disturbance in the category of *higher cerebral functions,* suggesting that lesions are at the highest level of motor integration in the nervous system (Kirshner, 1986). In adults, actual lesions generally have been localized to the left hemisphere at a cortical level or at immediate subcortical areas (Kertesz, 1984; Tognola & Vignolo, 1980). The assumption is generally held that similar disturbances in children are also at the highest level of motor integration, but to date, the limited neurologic evidence supporting this view is highly controversial (Darwish, Pearce, Gaines, & Harasym, 1982; Horwitz, 1984). In contrast to the verbal and oral dyspraxias, lesions in both child and adult dysarthria are, for the most part, at lower motor integration levels in the nervous system (Darley et al., 1975). In fact, Lenneberg (1967, p. 64) speculated years ago that this is particularly true in children.

Psycholinguistic theory of speech motor control does not concern itself with disorders and sites of lesion, but it does provide models of speech processes necessary for speech motor control. In Levett's (1989) model, motor planning and programming are at an early stage of the speech motor process of speaking, while motor execution is at a later stage.

Combining the salient features of these two theoretical models, there are useful contrasts that can be drawn between childhood dysarthria and DVD. Childhood dysarthria is likely to be a disorder of motor execution occurring at late stages in the motor speech processes in which lesions are generally at lower levels of the nervous system. In contrast, developmental verbal dyspraxia is likely to be a disorder of motor planning and programming in which normal processing occurs at an early stage of speech motor control. It is assumed lesions are at higher levels of the nervous system. Of course, only future research will confirm the validity of these heuristic theoretical distinctions, but in the meantime, communication specialists may find them helpful when dealing with what are considered confusing features of childhood motor speech problems.

CHARACTERISTICS OF CHILDHOOD DYSARTHRIA

Our understanding of dysarthrias in children has a long history. As seen in the chapter epigraph by Dr. William J. Little, the classic description of the disorder in cerebral palsy achieved worldwide attention in the medical literature almost 150 years ago. Reports of speech problems of dysarthric children, primarily centering on cerebral palsy, have been appearing in the American speech-pathology literature for well over half a century.

In contrast, modern attention was first called to the syndrome of DVD in the 1950s (Morley, 1957; Morley, Court, Miller, & Garside, 1955), but widespread interest in this developmental communication disorder in the United States did not develop until the 1970s (Chappell, 1973; Daly, Cantrell, Cantrell, & Aman, 1972; Darley & Spriestersbach, 1978; Edwards, 1973; Emerick & Hatten, 1979; Ferry, Hall, & Hicks, 1975; Kools, Williams, Vickers, & Caell, 1971; Malcaluso-Haynes, 1978; Pritchard, Tekieli, & Kozup, 1977; Rosenbek, Hansen, Baugham, & Lemme, 1974; Rosenbek & Wertz, 1972; Smartt, LaLance, Gray, & Hibbett, 1976; Yoss & Darley, 1974a, b).

The characteristics of this syndrome have been seriously questioned (Guyette & Diedrich, 1981); the only commercial test for the disorder has been sharply criticized and condemned (Guyette & Diedrich, 1983; Thompson, 1988); and the validity of diagnosis has been challenged (Love & Fitzgerald, 1984; Thompson, 1988). It is clearly the consensus of most speech and language pathologists that the disorder is controversial on many levels and that there is little agreement on its characteristics. This issue is so controversial, in fact, that a whole chapter—Chapter 5—is devoted to its characteristics.

Age of Onset

Childhood dysarthrias are characterized as **congenital disorders** or **acquired disorders** in terms of whether the underlying cause of the dysarthria was a disease present at birth or one that had an onset later in the pediatric period (0–15 years). Examples of common congenital dysarthrias are those of the cerebral palsies and of the Moebius syndrome. Frequently, these dysarthrias are classified as developmental because they emerge as the child matures (Ingram, 1969).

Acquired dysarthrias have their onset in a pediatric time frame but are distinguished from congenital and developmental problems by a period of normal speech and language development and normal school performance. Limited reports are available on acquired dysarthrias in children. In one of the few reports, van Dongen, Arts, and Yousef-Bak (1987) have observed that the site of lesion (central versus peripheral) is critical in the severity and recovery of the acquired dysarthrias of childhood.

Etiology

Dworkin and Hartman (1988) have presented a useful classification for the general causes of adult neurogenic communication disorders. The system is also useful for classifying the several causes of childhood dysarthria. The categories include (1) vascular, (2) infectious, (3) traumatic/toxic, (4) anoxic, (5) metabolic, (6) idiopathic, (7) neoplastic, and (8) degenerative/demyelinating. Dworkin and Hartman suggest using the acronym *Vitamin-D* as a mnemonic device for recalling the classification categories.

The etiologies of the most frequent childhood condition associated with dysarthria—cerebral palsy—have been studied extensively. Prematurity, anoxia, injury of brain due to mechanical factors, intrauterine infection and kernicterus are the more common causes of cerebral palsy; however, almost 50% of the cases present no obvious etiology, since there are no clear-cut perinatal complications (Erenberg, 1984). In some cases, genetic disorders are also causative of childhood dysarthria, including Duchenne muscular dystrophy, Huntington's disease, familial dysautonomia, cerebral palsy, and so forth. Closed head injury is a common cause of acquired dysarthria in children.

Site of Lesion

Site of lesion is an important characteristic of the dysarthrias both in children and in adults, because the concept is the basis for most current classifications of dysarthria. The most widely used site-of-lesion classification of the dysarthrias is known as the Mayo Clinic classification system. It is an empirically derived classification, but it is based entirely on research of dysarthric adults (Darley, Aronson, & Brown, 1969a, b; 1975); for instance, distinctive dysarthric patterns are reported for Parkinson's disease and multiple sclerosis (Aronson, 1981). These diseases, however, are not seen in childhood. The system includes six dysarthrias: flaccid, spastic, ataxic, hypokinetic, hyperkinetic, and mixed.

Espir and Rose (1983) have presented a site-of-lesion classification for the childhood dysarthrias that is based on classic sites of lesion presented in the clinical literature of neurology. Five major sites are included: (1) muscle, (2) lower motor neuron, (3) upper motor neuron, (4) extrapyramidal, and (5) cerebellar.

When dysarthria is associated with a muscle disorder such as muscular dystrophy, a flaccid dysarthria with articulation deficits predominates. Lower motor neuron disorders are associated with a childhood bulbar palsy, which includes diseases such as Bell palsy, Moebius syndrome, and anterior bulbar poliomyelitis. Flaccid dysarthria with misarticulation or misarticulation and hypernasality occurs. Upper motor neuron disorders are associated with congenital suprabulbar paresis. The cranial nerves V, VII, IX, X, XI, and

XII are usually affected to varying degrees. A spastic dysarthria results with several abnormal articulatory and vocal features. This syndrome may be part of a spastic diplegia or spastic quadriplegia of cerebral palsy.

Extrapyramidal lesion sites are associated with a spectrum of movement disorders in children, which include chorea, athetosis, choreoathetosis, dystonia, and tremor. These disorders all produce complex and often severe dysarthrias. Espir and Rose do not provide an inclusive term to describe the dysarthrias associated with extrapyramidal sites, but others have used terms common in neurology to describe these movement disorders. Darley et al. (1975) have labeled these dysarthrias hyperkinetic. Canter (1967) and Love and Webb (1996) have employed the term dyskinetic dysarthria. Cerebellar disorders result in ataxic dysarthria. Espir and Rose do not include the concept of mixed dysarthrias. This is a serious oversight since it is typical to have multiple involvement of motor systems in childhood neurologic impairment.

Although Espir and Rose's system is similar to the widely used Mayo Clinic classification system, some speech experts (Stark, 1985) have reservations about its use in children. First, empirical research has not yet completely supported distinctive speech patterns in all the developmental dysarthrias. Second, there is also the problem of using terms like spastic dysarthria, flaccid dysarthria, dyskinetic dysarthria, extrapyramidal dysarthria, ataxic dysarthria, and so forth. These labels, as noted earlier, are based on classic descriptions of disorders of limb and trunk involvement in the neurologic examination rather than demonstrated disorders of oral involvement in neurologically impaired children. The terms may not exactly be appropriate for the oromotor involvement in childhood dysarthria.

Another site-of-lesion classification system employs a more neuroanatomic approach than does the clinical classification system of Espir and Rose (1983), which really is a blend of both neuroanatomy and neurophysiology. This system divides the nervous system into its central and peripheral components as well as its structural divisions: (1) cerebrum, (2) cerebellum, (3) basal ganglia, (4) brain stem, (5) cranial nerve, and (6) spinal cord. This classification system has features that enhance our understanding of childhood dysarthria but may not be as useful as a Mayo Clinic or Espir and Rose classification system. At present, the following list may be the most useful clinical classification outline for the childhood dysarthrias: (1) spastic, (2) dyskinetic, (3) ataxic, (4) flaccid, and (5) mixed.

Primary Neurologic Disease

All childhood dysarthrias are considered medically to be a secondary symptom of a primary neurologic disease or condition. These diseases or conditions can be classified broadly as those of the central nervous system or peripheral nervous system. (See Chapters 3 and 4.) The cerebral palsies are a major group of disorders of the central nervous system. Disorders of the peripheral nervous system encompass a wide spectrum of diseases and neurologic conditions. Included are Werdnig-Hoffmann disease, progressive bulbar palsy, Moebius syndrome, Bell palsy, vocal cord paralysis, familial dysautomina, Duchenne muscular dystrophy, myotonic dystrophy, myopathies, and so forth.

At times, both speech-language pathologists and physicians have classified dysarthria as a symptom of a primary disease. Reports by speech-language pathologists of Moebius syndrome and its speech and hearing characteristics are typical of the classification of childhood dysarthria by disease (Kahane, 1979; Meyerson & Fourshee, 1978). Fenichel (1997), a pediatric neurologist, cites the presence or absence of childhood dysarthria with major diseases described in his comprehensive textbook survey of pediatric neurologic problems, but does not classify the dysarthria by the Mayo Clinic, Espir and Rose or neuroanatomic systems. Instead, Fenichel classifies dysarthria as a symptom of a primary disease only.

In brief, understanding the characteristics of the underlying primary neurologic disease frequently allows a better understanding of the childhood dysarthria associated with it, and it is an approach that is appealing to physicians.

Cranial Nerves

A significant characteristic of childhood dysarthrias is cranial nerve involvement. Six of the twelve paired cranial nerves contribute to motor speech production. The cranial nerves act as a final common pathway in the nervous system and reflect normal and abnormal motor integration at all levels above the level of the cranial nerves. The traditional peripheral oral examination that the speech-language pathologist usually performs can be viewed as an extended cranial nerve examination for the six cranial nerves of speech. These nerves are trigeminal (V), facial (VII), glossopharyngeal (IX), vagus (X), spinal accessory (XI), and hypoglossal (XII). The evaluation process described in Chapter 7 discusses cranial nerve assessment.

Speech Motor Processes

One or more of the basic processes of motor speech may be disturbed to varying degrees in childhood dysarthria. These processes involve respiratory, phonatory, velopharyngeal, and articulatory muscle systems. Guidelines for systematic assessment of these processes are presented in Chapter 7. If the technology of the modern speech laboratory is available, sophisticated assessment of the interactions of these motor speech processes can be made (Netsell, Lotz, & Barlow, 1989).

Natural Course

The childhood dysarthrias generally follow a predictable course. The developmental dysarthrias of cerebral palsy evolve until adulthood when there is a stabilization of the speech pattern (Platt, Andrews, Young, & Quinn, 1980). In contrast, the degenerative dysarthria of Duchenne muscular dystrophy shows a period of normal speech development, then a rapid decline of speech as the child reaches the terminal stages of the disease (Sanders & Perlstein, 1965). Children who have sustained closed head injury with dysarthric symptoms usually show improvement for at least two years post-insult (Stark, 1985). There are, however, variations in the natural course of some dysarthrias. Nelson and Ellenberg (1982) report that some cerebral-palsied children who have neurologic signs at birth show resolution of these signs by 7 years of age. This transient cerebral palsy group, however, displays persisting articulatory abnormality without any specific deviant motor signs when the lips, tongue, and pharynx are examined. Acquired childhood dysarthria displays a specific natural course of a speedier recovery in peripheral than in central dysarthria (van Dongen, Arts, & Yousef-Bak, 1987).

Predisposing Factors

Children with central or peripheral congenital dysarthria often have a history of infantile dysphagia and abnormal development of oral reflexes. Severity of the dysphagic symptoms in cerebral palsy usually predicts future dysarthria better than do abnormal oral reflexes (Love, Hagerman, & Tiami, 1980; Neilson & O'Dwyer, 1981).

Severity

Childhood dysarthria ranges in severity from complete lack of speech, or anarthria, to a disorder so mild that it may be confused either with a resolving developmental phonologic disorder or a developmental verbal dyspraxia. In confusion such as this, birth histories of hypoxia, periventricular hemorrhage, or jaundice would suggest possible central dysarthria rather than either a developmental phonologic disorder or verbal dyspraxia.

SUMMARY

Childhood motor speech disability includes the childhood dysarthrias and developmental verbal dyspraxia. Childhood dysarthria is defined as a neurogenic speech impairment caused by dysfunction of the motor control centers of the immature brain and is marked by disturbances of the speech muscles in speed, strength, steadiness, coordination, precision, tone, and range of motion. In contrast, developmental verbal dyspraxia is defined as an impaired ability to execute voluntarily the expected motor program for articulation in the absence of obvious muscular disturbance of the speech mechanism. Generally, in DVD the speech gestures cannot be performed voluntarily, but the movements can be performed automatically on a nonspeech level. A condition called developmental oral apraxia may or may not accompany DVD. This is an inability to perform nonspeech movements of the pharynx, tongue, and lips voluntarily or on command even though these movements may be maintained on a more automatic level in chewing and swallowing.

The study of the childhood dysarthrias has a long history, and there is a general consensus as to their nature and significant characteristics. DVD has had a much shorter history, and there is dispute as to its nature and defining characteristics. It is generally considered to be controversial as a diagnosis on several levels.

Childhood dysarthrias are classified as congenital (developmental) or acquired. Differences in severity and speed of recovery vary with age of onset of the underlying disease and the dysarthria. Dysarthrias in children have been generally classified according to primary neurologic disease, etiology, and site of lesion. Site-of-lesion classifications combined with associated motor symptoms are popular among speech-language pathologists for classifying the adult dysarthrias but have not been as widely accepted in classifying the childhood dysarthrias. However, spastic (upper motor neuron disorder), dyskinetic (basal ganglia disorder), ataxic (cerebellar disorder), flaccid (lower motor neuron disorder), and mixed dysarthrias (multiple motor system disorder) may serve as a workable classification system until empirical speech data are available to revise the classification system for children.

Varying cranial nerve involvement is common in the childhood dysarthrias, and cranial nerves V, VII, IX, X, XI, and XII are critical. The motor speech disorder in dysarthria can be understood by assessing the muscular subsystems that support the basic processes of speech. The speech processes include the functions of the respiratory, phonatory, velopharyngeal, and articulatory musculature. The natural course of the various childhood dysarthrias and severity of the speech disorder are important considerations in management and recovery of the dysarthric child.

SUGGESTED READING

Darley, F. L., Aronson, A. E., & Brown, J. R. (1975). *Motor speech disorders.* Philadelphia: W. B. Sanders.

This book has become a modern classic in defining the concept of adult motor speech disorders and provides the basis for understanding childhood motor speech disability.

Duffy, J. R. (1995). *Motor speech disorders.* St. Louis, MO: Mosby-Yearbook.

This is an excellent current text on diagnosis and management of adult motor speech disability.

Jaffe, M. B. (1986). Neurologic impairment of speech production: Assessment and treatment. In J. M. Costello, & A. L. Holland (Eds.), *Handbook of speech and language disorders* (pp. 157–186). San Diego: College Hill Press.

This chapter discusses pertinent current issues related to childhood dysarthria and developmental verbal dyspraxia.

Stark, R. E. (1985). Dysarthria in children. In J. B. Darby (Ed.), *Speech and language evaluation in neurology: Childhood disorders* (pp. 185–217). New York: Grune & Stratton.

This serves as an excellent critical review of the topic of childhood dysarthria.

Yorkston, K. M., Beukelman, D. R., Strand, E. A., & Bell, K. R. (1999). *Management of motor speech disorders in children and adults* (2nd ed.). Austin, TX: Pro-ed.

A recent book of diagnosis and management of motor speech disorders.

REFERENCES

Abbs, J. H., Hunker, J. C., & Barlow, S. M. (1983). Differential speech motor subsystem impairments with suprabulbar lesions: Neurophysiological framework and supporting data. In W. Berry (Ed.), *Clinical dysarthria.* San Diego, CA: College Hill Press.

Aram, D. M., & Nation, J. E. (1982). *Child language disorders.* St. Louis, MO: C. V. Mosby.

Aronson, A. E. (1981). Motor speech signs of neurologic disease. In J. K. Darby, Jr. (Ed.), *Speech evaluation in medicine.* New York: Grune & Stratton.

Bayley, N. (1969). *Bayley Scales of Infant Development.* New York: Psychological Corp.

Bishop, D. V. M. (1988). Language development in children with abnormal structure or function of the speech apparatus. In D. V. M. Bishop & K. Mogford (Eds.), *Language development in exceptional circumstances* (pp. 220–238). Edinburgh, Great Britain: Churchill Livingstone.

Bishop, D. V. M., Brown, B. B., & Robson, J. (1990). The relationship between phoneme discrimination, speech production and language comprehension in cerebral-palsied individuals. *Journal of Speech and Hearing Research, 33,* 210–219.

Buckingham, H. W., Jr. (1981). Explanations for the concept of apraxia of speech. In M. T. Sarno (Ed.), *Acquired aphasia* (pp. 271–301). New York: Academic Press.

Canter, G. J. (1967). Neuromotor pathologies of speech. *American Journal of Physical Medicine, 46,* 659–666.

Chappell, G. (1973). Childhood verbal apraxia and its treatment. *Journal of Speech and Hearing Disorders, 38,* 362–368.

Charcot, J. M. (1877). *Lectures on the diseases of the nervous system* (Vol. 1). London: The New Sydenham Society.

Daly, D. A., Cantrell, R. P., Cantrell, M. L., & Aman, L. A. (1972). Structuring speech therapy contingencies with an oral apraxic child. *Journal of Speech and Hearing Disorders, 37,* 22–32.

Darley, F. L., Aronson, A. E., & Brown, J. R. (1969a). Differential diagnostic patterns of dysarthria. *Journal of Speech & Hearing Research, 12,* 246–269.

Darley, F. L., Aronson, A. E., & Brown, J. R. (1969b). Clusters of deviant speech dimensions in the dysarthrias. *Journal of Speech & Hearing Research, 12,* 462–496.

Darley, F. L., Aronson, A. E., & Brown, J. E. (1975). *Motor speech disorders.* Philadelphia: W. B. Saunders.

Darley, F. L., & Spriestersbach, D. C. (1978). *Diagnostic methods in speech pathology* (2nd ed.). New York: Harper.

Darwish, H., Pearce, P. S., Gaines, R., & Harasym, P. (1982). The speech programming deficit syndrome. *Annals of Neurology, 12,* 21.

DeRenzi, E., Pieczuro, A., & Vignolo, L. A. (1966). Oral apraxia and aphasia. *Cortex, 2,* 749–756.

Duffy, J. R. (1995). *Motor speech disorders.* St. Louis, MO: Mosby-Yearbook.

Dworkin, J. P., & Hartman, D. E. (1988). *Cases in neurogenic comrnunicative disorders.* Boston: Little, Brown.

Edwards, M. (1973). Developmental verbal dyspraxia. *British Journal of Communication Disorders, 8,* 64–70.

Emerick, L. L., & Hatten, J. T. (1979). *Diagnosis and evaluation in speech pathology* (2nd ed.). Englewood Cliffs, NJ: Prentice Hall.

Erenberg, G. (1984). Cerebral palsy. *Postgraduate Medicine, 75,* 87–93.

Espir, M. L. E., & Rose, F. C. (1983). *The basic neurology of speech* (3rd ed.). Philadelphia: F. A. Davis.

Fenichel, G. M. (1997). *Clinical pediatric neurology* (3rd ed.). Philadelphia: W. B. Saunders.

Ferry, P. C., Hall, S. M., & Hicks, J. L. (1975). 'Dilapidated' speech: Developmental verbal apraxia. *Developmental Medicine and Child Neurology, 17,* 749–756.

Fisher, H. B., & Logemann, J. A. (1971). *Fisher-Logemann Test of Articulation Competence.* Boston: Houghton Mifflin.

Flower, R. M., Viehweg, R., & Ruzicka, W. R. (1966). The communicative disorders of children with Kernicteric athetosis: Problems in language comprehension and use. *Journal of Speech and Hearing Disorders, 31,* 60–68.

Goldman, R., Fristoe, M., & Woodcock, R. A. (1974). *Goldman-Fristoe-Woodcock Auditory Skills Battery.* Circle Pines, MN: American Guidance Service.

Guyette, T. W., & Diedrich, W. R. (1981). A critical review of developmental apraxia of speech. In N. Lass (Ed.), *Speech and language: Advances in basic research and practice* (Vol. 1, pp. 1–49). New York: Academic Press.

Guyette, T. W., & Diedrich, W. A. (1983). A review of the Screening Test for Developmental Apraxia of Speech. *Language, Speech, and Services in Schools, 14,* 202–209.

Hier, D. B., Gorelick, P. D., & Shindler, A. G. (1987). *Topics in behavioral neurology and neuropsychology.* Boston: Butterworth.

Horwitz, S. J. (1984). Neurological findings in developmental verbal apraxia. *Seminars in Speech and Language, 5,* 111–118.

Ingram, T. T. S. (1969). Developmental disorders of speech. In P. J. Vinken & G. W. Bruyn (Eds.), *Handbook of clinical neurology* (Vol. 4). Amsterdam: North Holland.

Jastak, J. F. (1965). *Wide Range Achievement Test.* Wilmington, VA: Guidance Associates.

Kahane, J. (1979). Pathophysiological effect of Moebius syndrome on speech and hearing. *Archives of Otolaryngology, 105,* 29–34.

Kertesz, A. (1984). Subcortical lesions and verbal apraxia. In J. C. Rosenbek, M. R. McNeil, & A. E. Aronson (Eds.), *Apraxia of speech: Physiology-acoustics-linguistics-management*. San Diego, CA: College Hill Press.

Kirshner, H. S. (1986). *Behavioral neurology: A practical approach*. Edinburgh: Churchill Livingstone.

Kools, J. A., Williams, A. F., Vickers, M. J., & Caell, A. (1971). Oral and limb apraxia in mentally retarded children with defective articulation. *Cortex, 7,* 387–400.

Koppitz, E. M. (1964). *The Bender Gestalt Test for Children*. New York: Psychological Corp.

Leipmann, H. (1908). *Drei Aufsatze dem Apraxiegebeit* (Vol. 1). Berlin: Krager.

Lenneberg, E. (1967). *Biological foundations of language*. New York: John Wiley.

Levett, W. J. M. (1989). *Speaking: From intention to articulation*. Cambridge, MA: MIT Press.

Little, W. J. (1861). On the influence of abnormal parturition, difficult labour, premature birth, and asphyxia neonatorum on the mental and physical condition of the child, especially in relation to deformities. *Lancet, 2,* 378–380.

Love, R. J. (1964). Oral language behavior of older cerebral palsied children. *Journal of Speech and Hearing Research, 7,* 349–359.

Love, R. J., & Fitzgerald, M. (1984). Is the diagnosis of developmental apraxia of speech valid? *Australian Journal of Human Communication Disorders, 12,* 71–82.

Love, R. J., Hagerman, E. L., & Tiami, E. G. (1980). Speech performance, dysphagia and oral reflexes in cerebral palsy. *Journal of Speech and Hearing Disorders, 45,* 59–75.

Love, R. J., & Webb, W. G. (1996). *Neurology for the speech-language pathologist* (3rd ed.). Boston: Butterworth.

Malcaluso-Haynes, S. (1978). Developmental apraxia of speech: Symptoms and treatment. In D. F. Johns (Ed.), *Clinical management of neurogenic communicative disorders* (pp. 243–250). Boston: Little, Brown.

Meyerson, M., & Fourchee, D. (1978). Speech, language and hearing in Moebius syndrome. *Developmental Medicine and Child Neurology, 20,* 357–365.

Morley, M. E. (1957). *The development and disorders of speech in childhood* (1st ed.). London: Livingstone.

Morley, M., Court, D., Miller, H., & Garside, R. (1955). Delayed speech and developmental aphasia. *British Medical Journal, 2,* 463–467.

Myers, P. (1965). A study of language disabilities in cerebral palsied children. *Journal of Speech and Hearing Research, 8,* 129–136.

Neilson, P. D., & O'Dwyer, N. J. (1981). Pathophysiology of dysarthria in cerebral palsy. *Journal of Neurology, Neurosurgery and Psychiatry, 44,* 1013–1019.

Nelson, K. B., & Ellenberg, J. H. (1982). Children who "outgrew" cerebral palsy. *Pediatrics, 69,* 529–536.

Netsell, R., Lotz, W. K., & Barlow, S. M. (1989). A speech physiology examination for individuals with dysarthria. In K. M. Yorkston & D. R. Beukelman (Eds.), *Recent advances in clinical dysarthria* (pp. 3–37). Boston: Little, Brown.

Platt, L., Andrews, G., Young, M., & Quinn, P. T. (1980). Dysarthria of adult cerebral palsy: 1. Intelligibility and articulatory impairment. *Journal of Speech and Hearing Research, 23,* 22–40.

Pritchard, C. L., Tekieli, M. E., & Kozup, J. M. (1977). Developmental apraxia: Diagnostic considerations. *Journal of Communication Disorders, 12,* 337–348.

Rosenbek, J., Hansen, R., Baugham, C., & Lemme, M. (1974). Treatment of developmental apraxia of speech: A case study. *Language, Speech and Hearing Services in Schools, 5,* 13–22.

Rosenbek, J., & Wertz, R. (1972). A review of 50 cases of developmental apraxia of speech. *Language, Speech, and Hearing Services in Schools, 3,* 23–33.

Sanders, L. J., & Perlstein, M. A. (1965). Speech mechanism in pseudohyperthrophic muscular dystrophy. *American Journal of Diseases of Children, 109,* 538–543.

Smartt, J., LaLance, L., Gray, J., & Hibbett, P. (1976). Developmental apraxia: A Tennessee Speech and Hearing Association subcommittee report. *Journal of the Tennessee Speech and Hearing Association, 20,* 21–39.

Stark, R. E. (1985). Dysarthria in children. In J. K. Darby, Jr. (Ed.), *Speech and language in neurology: Childhood disorders* (pp. 185–217). New York: Grune & Stratton.

Terman, L. M., & Merrill, M. A. (1973). *Manual for the third revision (Form L-M) of the Stanford-Binet Intelligence Scale.* Boston: Houghton Mifflin.

Thompson, C. K.(1988). Articulation disorders in the child with neurogenic pathology. In N. J. Lass, L. V. McReynolds, J. L. Northern, & D. E. Yoder (Eds.), *Handbook of speech-language pathology and audiology* (pp. 548–591). Toronto: B. C. Decker.

Tiegs, E. W., & Clark, W. W. (1957). *California Achievement Test.* Los Angeles: California Test Bureau.

Tognola, G., & Vignolo, L. A. (1980). Brain lesions associated with oral apraxia in stroke patients: A cliniconeuroradiological investigation with CT scan. *Neuropsychologica, 18,* 257–262.

van Dongen, H. R., Arts, W. F. M., & Yousef-Bak, E. (1987). Acquired dysarthria in childhood: An analysis of dysarthric features in relation to neurologic deficits. *Neurology, 37,* 296–299.

Wechsler, D. (1974). *Wechsler Intelligence Scale for Children-Revised.* New York: Psychological Corp.

Wertz, R. T., LaPointe, L. L., & Rosenbek, J. C. (1984). *Apraxia of speech in adults: The disorder and its management.* New York: Grune & Stratton.

Wiig, E., & Semmel, E. (1980). *Clinical Evaluation of Language Function.* Columbus, OH: Merrill.

Yorkston, K. M., Beukelman, D. R., Strand, E. A., & Bell, K. R. (1999). *Management of motor speech disorders in children and adults.* Austin, TX: Pro-ed.

Yoss, K. A., & Darley, F. L. (1974a). Developmental apraxia of speech in children with defective articulation. *Journal of Speech and Hearing Research, 17,* 339–416.

Yoss, K. A., & Darley, F. L. (1974b). Therapy in developmental apraxia of speech. *Language, Speech and Hearing Services in Schools, 5,* 23–31.

► 2

The Neurology of Childhood Motor Speech Disability

Acoustically distinct disorders of motor speech reflect discrete nervous dysfunctions. This fact is of practical clinical usefulness, of course, but it also teaches important information about the nervous system's working.
—FREDERIC L. DARLEY, ARNOLD E. ARONSON,
AND JOE R. BROWN, 1975

The Motor System

Cortical Level
  Motor Functions • Speech Control

Descending Motor Pathways
  Direct Motor System

Subcortical Level
  Indirect Motor System

Peripheral Motor System Pathways
  Final Common Pathway • Cranial Nerves for Speech

Clinical Neurology of the Childhood Dysarthrias
  Upper Motor Neuron Lesions: Spasticity • Lower Motor Neuron Lesions: Flaccidity • Basal Ganglia Lesions: Dyskinesia • Cerebellum and Cerebellar Pathway Lesions: Ataxia

Clinical Neurology of Developmental Verbal Dyspraxia
Evidence of Brain Dysfunction

THE MOTOR SYSTEM

Speech-language pathologists who elect to study and treat childhood motor speech disabilities must understand the functions and dysfunctions of the human motor system. Integration of motor speech requires the interaction of the three major motor subsystems—the pyramidal system, nasal ganglia system, and cerebellar system—at several levels in the nervous system. Five levels can be identified: (1) cortical level, (2) subcortical level of the basal ganglia, (3) brain-stem level, (4) cerebellar level, and (5) spinal level.

CORTICAL LEVEL

Motor Functions

The cerebral cortex contains motor and sensory areas that are critical to the normal performance of skilled voluntary movements. Three functional stages are likely to occur in the motor control of skilled movement: motor planning, motor programming, and motor execution (McClean, 1988). These stages are reflected in the functions of the various cortical motor areas, as we know them so far. The primary or somatic motor area (Area 4), also known as the motor strip, is located in the precentral gyrus of the frontal lobe (Figure 2-1). This area is involved to a great extent in the execution stage of motor performance. The area serves to activate motor neurons, muscle contractions, and voluntary movements. The motor strip is bilateral, found in both cerebral hemispheres. The right motor strip controls the left side of the body and the left strip controls the right side. The tongue and larynx are controlled by neurons in the lowest part of the dual motor strips. They are followed in an ascending order along the strips by the face, thumb, forearm, arm, thorax, abdomen, thigh, leg, and foot areas. The areas for the tongue and larynx, as well as the hand, are disproportionately large. These large areas, which are given over to motor control of the oral mechanism, promote the rapid and precise movements demanded during speaking and singing activities.

A second motor area is known as the premotor area (lateral Area 6 and Area 8). This area is considered a supplement to the primary motor area. Area 6 integrates movements of the body musculature, and Area 8 influences eye movements. Specifically, Area 6 is involved in the motor planning and motor programming stages of motor control. The area has extensive inter-

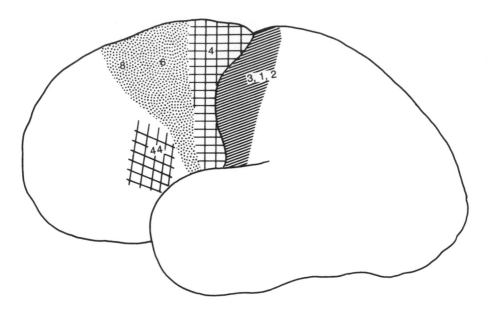

FIGURE 2-1   Cortical Motor Areas Involved in Speech Control
Area 4 is the primary motor cortex. Areas 3, 1, and 2 are the somatosensory cortex. Areas 6 and 8 make up the premotor cortex and the supplementary motor areas. Area 44 is Broca's area.

connections with Area 4, and it is generally believed that Area 6 serves to shape the motor output of Area 4.

Another motor area of importance is the supplementary motor area (medial Area 6). Its function is not completely understood, but it is thought to be involved in the motor planning and programming of sequential and complex movements, such as simultaneous limb movements on both sides of the body. The supplementary motor area also has extensive connections with Area 4.

Lesions of Area 4 produce muscle weakness and are correlated with muscle changes in learned movements. If both Area 4 and Area 6 are ablated, spasticity occurs in the limbs.

Speech Control

The classic motor planning and programming area for speech is Broca's area (Area 44). It is located in the frontal lobe anterior to the lower end of the motor strip and can be considered a motor association area for the primary motor area. The cytoarchitecture of Area 44 is similar in both the left and right hemispheres, but traditional neurologic theory maintains that the left hemisphere is involved primarily in motor speech formulation. Regional cerebral blood flow (CBF) and cerebral metabolic rate (CMR) studies have suggested that both these right and left cortical areas may be activated during some speech functions, but activity is greater in the left cortical areas in most persons (Ingvar, 1983). However, motor planning and programming of oral motor activities may not be the exclusive province of the motor areas in the frontal lobe. Mateer and Kimura (1977) have reported oral movement sequencing disorders in some aphasic adults with lesions in the posterior perisylvian cortex as well as oral motor problems in traditional anterior locations of the frontal lobe in the perisylvian cortex. This suggests that, at least in adults, there may be more than one site in the cortex for the oral motor planning and programming that underlie speech activity.

Although there is considerable agreement that lesions in, around, or deep to Broca's area in the left hemisphere are predominately associated with oral and verbal praxic symptoms in adults, there is no evidence as yet that children diagnosed with developmental verbal dyspraxia and/or oral dyspraxia present the same classic features of lateralization and localization of lesions that are found in adults diagnosed with dyspraxic symptoms. Further, developmental neuroanatomy and neurophysiology research has not yet provided significant information to aid in understanding developmental dyspraxic symptoms. The only fact that might lead to speculation about this issue is that the triangular gyrus, which becomes Broca's area in the adult brain, first shows formation and definition around the 28th week of gestation. Unlike the primary motor and sensory areas of the cortex, which myelinate early, Broca's convolution is one of the last areas of the cortex to mature (Bunger, 1989). It is not clear whether a disturbance or delay in this particular developmental schedule of myelination contributes to dyspraxic disorders in children.

DESCENDING MOTOR PATHWAYS

Direct Motor System

The descending motor pathways of the nervous system include both direct and indirect fiber tracts that project to various levels of the system. The direct motor system is often called the pyramidal tract or system. The pyramidal pathway was once believed to be the pathway that initiated all voluntary movement, but it is now considered to be concerned primarily with the skilled movements of the limbs and digits as well as innervating special motor neurons (alpha and gamma motor neurons) that control the flexor muscles of the limbs. The pyramidal system is a direct motor system, because the motor tracts of which it is composed originate in the motor cortex and descend directly, without synapsing, to the brain stem or spinal cord, thus allowing rapid motor voluntary response when needed.

Corticospinal and Corticobulbar Tracts.   The pyramidal system is subdivided into the corticospinal tract and the corticobulbar tract (Figure 2-2). The latter tract is important in speech production. The corticobulbar tract arises from neurons in the ventral lateral part of Areas 4 and 6 and Area 8. The corticobulbar fibers descend in company with corticospinal fibers to the midbrain level in the brain stem where they take divergent routes to terminate in the lower brain stem on the motor nuclei of the cranial nerves. The corticobulbar system does not go beyond the inferior border of the medulla oblongata (bulb). This system is critical to motor speech activity since it directly influences the actions of motor cranial nerves that innervate oral musculature, including cranial nerves V (trigeminal), VII (facial), IX (glossopharyngeal), X (vagus), XI (accessory), and XII (hypoglossal). Lesions in the corticobulbar system produce a spastic dysarthria.

The corticospinal tract arises from various sensory-motor areas of the cerebral cortex. About a third of the fibers originate from Area 4 and only about 3% of these arise from the large pyramidal cells, called Betz cells, in the fifth cell layer of the cortex. Another one-third arise from Area 6 and the remainder of the fibers come from the postcentral somatosensory area (Areas 3, 1, and 2) in the parietal lobe. The tracts descend through the corona radiata, a mass of white matter composed of descending motor fibers and ascending sensory fibers, and then enter the internal capsule in the diencephalon, where the corticospinal fibers are concentrated into a small area of the internal capsule.

Next, the fibers enter the brain stem, descending through the cerebral peduncles of the midbrain, the anterior portion of the pons, and the pyramids of the medulla, from which the pyramidal tract derives its name (Figure 2-3). At the lower margin of the medulla, most of the fibers decussate (crossover) to the opposite side. Approximately 90% of the fibers cross at this level and descend through the spinal cord as the lateral corticospinal tract. This tract passes to all levels of the spinal cord to innervate the spinal nerves exiting from the spinal cord. The 10% of the corticospinal fibers that do not decussate at the lower margin of the medulla descend in the anterior funiculus of the cervical and upper thoracic cord as the anterior corticospinal tract. The corticospinal tract is not purely motor. It sends fibers to synapse on the interneurons of the spinal cord, thus influencing local reflex arcs and the cells where ascending sensory pathways originate.

Lesions of the direct motor system interrupt passage of information to the motor nuclei of the brain stem and spinal cord. These lesions cause weakness or paralysis of the muscles innervated by the portion of the tract involved. Lesions of the system are **upper motor neuron disorders (UMN),** a

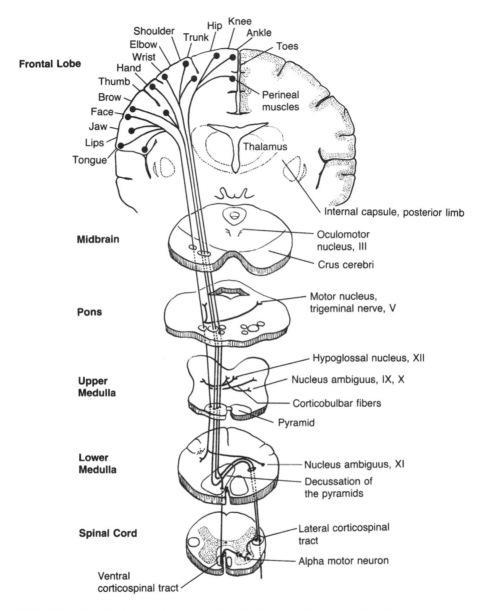

FIGURE 2-2   Corticospinal and Corticobulbar Tracts of the Central Nervous System

term usually used by physicians to describe the effect of lesions involving the corticospinal tract and the corticobulbar tract. **Lower motor neuron disorders (LMN),** in contrast, result from lesions that affect the motor neurons in

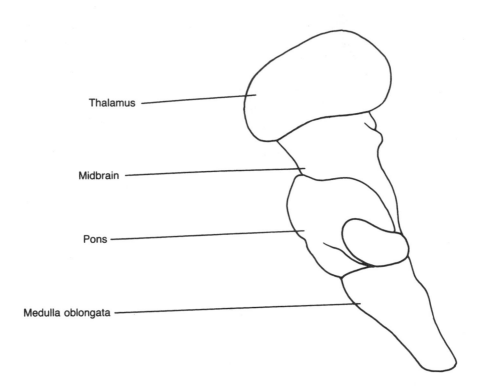

Thalamus

Midbrain

Pons

Medulla oblongata

FIGURE 2-3   The Four Transverse Subdivisions of the Brain Stem Shown in a Left Lateral View

the brain stem and spinal cord, the cranial and spinal nerves, their juncture with muscles (myoneural juncture), and the muscle itself. The motor neuron, the nerves, the junction with muscle, and the muscle fibers are a functional unit called the **motor unit.** Lesions at any point in the motor unit result in LMN disorders. They are associated with a flaccid dysarthria.

SUBCORTICAL LEVEL

Indirect Motor System

Subcortical motor systems of the basal ganglia and the cerebellum, along with their numerous and complex pathways, have a significant effect on movement by influencing the premotor and motor cortex. In the past, **extrapyramidal system** was the term used to describe all of the motor pathways that

TABLE 2-1   The Basal Ganglia System

Basal Ganglia

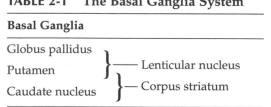

do not pass through the pyramids at the medullary-spinal cord juncture. The word *extrapyramidal,* however, has received sharp criticism on the grounds that it is inaccurate and inappropriate. Many neurologists prefer to use the term **basal ganglia** to refer to the subcortical nuclei and related pathways for the system, which, with the cerebellar system, interacts with the pyramidal system and affects the descending pathways of the direct motor system (Brodal, 1981; Weiner & Lang, 1989).

Basal Ganglia.   The interrelationships among the structures and circuits of the basal ganglia are complex, and the terminology used to describe the basal ganglia is confusing; but there is agreement on salient features (Table 2-1). The basal ganglia are a collection of large subcortical nuclei close to the thalamus, a midline brain-stem structure (Figure 2-4). It is likely that the basal ganglia make a special contribution to motor speech since several basal ganglia disorders present an accompanying dysarthria. The major components

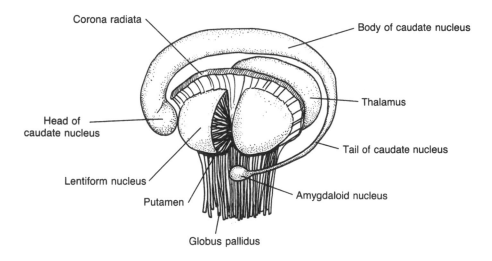

FIGURE 2-4   The Basal Ganglia and Adjacent Structures

of the basal ganglia include the **caudate nucleus,** the **putamen,** and the **globus pallidus.** The caudate nucleus and the putamen together are called the **corpus striatum.** The putamen and globus pallidus make up the **lenticular nucleus.** The substantia nigra and subthalamic nucleus, two other subcortical nuclei, are not part of the basal ganglia, per se, but are functionally related to it.

The basal ganglia has a complex series of connections with other components in the motor system. The striatum serves as the major receiving area of basal ganglia. Input comes from the cerebral cortex, the thalamus, and the substantia nigra, another subcortical nucleus that is not part of the basal ganglia proper.

The primary motor and sensory areas of the cortex project fibers particularly to the putamen. Fibers are projected to the caudate nucleus from the frontal, parietal, occipital, and temporal lobes. The neurons projecting from the cerebral cortex are excitatory and employ the neurotransmitter called glutamate. Neurons in the stratum project to the globus pallidus and are inhibitory in nature, using the neurotransmitter gamma-aminobutyric acid (GABA). Many of the interneurons of striatum are excitatory and use the neurotransmitter acetylcholine (Ach).

Output from the basal ganglia comes primarily from the globus pallidus. Fibers from the globus pallidus ascend to the level of the internal capsule where they join cerebellothalamic fibers and synapse in the thalamus. Other fibers from the globus pallidus synapse in the subthalamic nucleus, while another set terminate in the midbrain. There is a series of circuits and feedback loops between the corpus striatum, globus pallidus, thalamus, and cerebral cortex as well as circuits and a feedback loop involving the corpus striatum, substantia nigra, thalamus, and cerebral cortex. These two circuits ensure that the basal ganglia interacts with the cerebral cortex in all motor activity.

The functions of the basal ganglia are far from clear (Marsden, 1982), and it is difficult, from the results of lesions, to deduce its functions. Lesions of the basal ganglia have generally produced two major types of movement disorders: (1) poverty of movement (**akinesia**) and (2) excessive involuntary movement (**dyskinesia**) (Weiner & Lang, 1989). Akinesia is often accompanied by muscular rigidity (Parkinson's disease). The symptoms of these movement disorders have suggested that basal ganglia disease influences disorders of the initiation of movement (akinesia), difficulty in continuing or stopping an ongoing movement (dyskinesia), abnormalities of muscle tone (rigidity), and the development of involuntary movements (chorea, tremor, athetosis, dystonia). Thus the basal ganglia is thought to participate heavily in motor control, particularly in the initiation of movement, but also in the maintenance of ongoing movement. The basal ganglia particularly influences movements related to posture, automatic movements, and skilled voluntary movements.

Marsden (1982) argues that the basal ganglia are responsible for the automatic execution of learned motor plans. This involves the subconscious selection, sequencing, and delivery of the motor programs of a learned or practiced motor strategy, such as playing an instrument or handwriting. When the basal ganglia are damaged, it appears that the individual reverts to slower, less automatic, and less accurate, cortical mechanisms for motor behavior.

The effects of basal ganglia lesions are obvious, particularly in the speech mechanism. These lesions produce a dyskinetic dysarthria. The laryngeal system includes disorders such as breathiness, roughness, tremor, hoarseness, alteration of fundamental frequency control, and deficits in the ability to rapidly adduct and abduct the vocal folds in dyskinetic dysarthria (Barlow & Farley, 1989). Articulatory muscle control is also dramatically disturbed in basal ganglia disease. Exaggerated ranges of jaw movement, reduced range of tongue movement, instability of velar elevation, lip retrusion, and poor articulatory transitional movements are typical of dyskinetic dysarthria in athetosis (Kent & Netsell, 1978).

Cerebellum.   The cerebellum, like the basal ganglia, interacts with the cerebral cortex through a series of intricate circuits that ultimately influence the descending pathways of the direct motor system. In turn, these pathways affect the activity of the lower motor neurons. The cerebellum is located dorsal to the midbrain, pons, and medulla of the brain stem (Figure 2-5). The structure has two hemispheres connected by a midportion called the vermis. There are three cerebellar lobes: the anterior lobe, the posterior lobe, and the flocculonodular lobe. The cerebellum is connected to the brain stem by three rootlike structures called the cerebral peduncles. Afferent and efferent pathways transverse the peduncles to provide neural information to the remainder of the nervous system.

The cerebellum functions as a center for the control of coordinated movement and affects all stages of speech activity. The cerebellar cortex receives sensory input from the tongue, lips, jaw, larynx, and auditory system, and the information is integrated in the cerebellum for speech processing. Two major cerebellar pathways involving corticocerebellar circuits are important in cortical motor output for speech (McClean, 1988). One pathway involves Area-6 projections to the left cerebellar hemisphere through the pons, with a return pathway to cortical Areas 4 and 6 by way of deep cerebellar nuclei and ventral thalamic nuclei. This circuit involves planning and programming of learned movements. The second corticocerebellar pathway utilizes collateral projections of the descending corticospinal and corticobulbar pathways to the intermediate cerebellar hemisphere. This pathway provides the cerebellum with ongoing information on descending corticomotor output. The return path is to Area 4 from the intermediate cerebellar hemispheres through

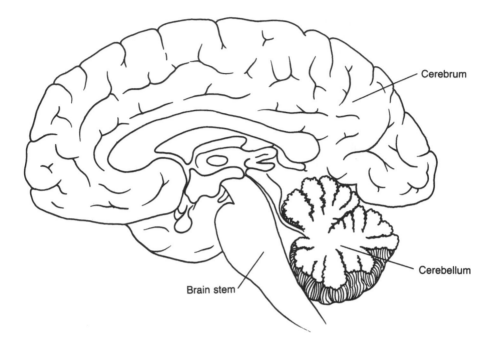

FIGURE 2-5   Medial View of the Cerebrum, Brain Stem, and Cerebellum

deep cerebellar nuclei and ventral thalamic nuclei. The intermediate hemispheres project to the brain stem and spinal cord via the red nucleus. It appears that the intermediate cerebellar hemispheres utilize sensory input to produce rapid changes of corticomotor output. It is likely then that a major function of the cerebellum is to provide coordination of rapid alternating movements, such as those required in speech.

Cerebellar damage results in a variety of signs, but decomposition of movement, dysmetria, dyssynergia, and ataxia are significant motor signs in adults. **Decomposition of movement** refers to the fact that various components of a motor act are performed in a jerky and irregular manner rather than in a smooth sequence. **Dysmetria** is the inability to gauge the distance, speed, and power of a movement. The movement may be stopped before the goal is reached, or the movement may overshoot the motor goal. **Dyssynergia** is a loss of coordination. **Ataxia** is a comprehensive term describing the problems in movement chiefly resulting from the effects of decomposition of movement, dyssynergia, and dysmetria. Errors in sequence and speed of the components of each movement characterize ataxia. *Nystagmus* (eye oscillations) and tremor with voluntary movement (*intention* or *action tremor*) are often present.

Dysarthria has been long recognized as a possible sign of ataxia in adults. The Mayo Clinic studies (Darley, Aronson, & Brown, 1975) of adult dysarthrics found that slowness of movements, hypotonia, and inaccuracy of repetitive movements lead to an ataxic dysarthria marked by excessive or equal stress, slowed rate, imprecise consonants, distorted vowels, mono-pitch, and monoloudness. The same speech symptoms appear in children.

PERIPHERAL MOTOR SYSTEM PATHWAYS

Final Common Pathway

The term **final common pathway** refers to the descending motor pathways of the peripheral nervous system. Specifically, these pathways involve the cranial and spinal nerves. The final common pathway, also known as the lower motor neuron (LMN), implies that the peripheral nerves serve as a last route in the nervous system, conveying neural information about the inter-actions of the direct and indirect motor systems to the muscles via the pe-ripheral nerves. In other words, neural messages summarizing the complex integration of the three major motor subsystems—pyramidal system, basal ganglia system, and cerebellar system—are transmitted via cranial and spinal nerves to activate the muscles of the body.

Cranial Nerves for Speech

As noted earlier, six of the twelve cranial nerves are important for motor pro-duction of speech. The final common pathways for motor speech involve cra-nial nerves V, VII, IX, X, XI, and XII. Table 2-2 lists the cranial motor nerves for speech and their major functions. Cranial nerves IX (glossopharyngeal), X (vagus), and XI (spinal-accessory) are bilaterally represented, innervating both ipsilateral and contralateral muscles of the speech mechanism. Cranial nerves V (trigeminal) and XII (hypoglossal) are primarily contralaterally in-nervated. Cranial nerve VII (facial) has mixed innervation. The upper face has both contralateral and ipsilateral innervation. The lower face is completely contralateral. This arrangement and innervation of cranial nerves is particu-larly important in understanding the consequences of an upper motor neu-ron (UMN) lesion. With unilateral UMN damage, cranial nerves IX, X, and XII remain unaffected because of their bilateral innervation. Mild and tran-sient contralateral involvement of the masticatory muscles (V) and tongue muscles (XII) usually occurs. The muscles of the lower face become para-lyzed, but the upper face generally remains intact. A mild or transient UMN dysarthria may result. With a bilateral UMN lesion, chronic spastic dysarthria and dysphagia (swallowing disorder) result. In LMN lesions of the cranial nerves, weakness of the innervated muscles occurs on the same side of the le-

TABLE 2-2   The Cranial Nerves and Their Functions

Number	Name	Summary of Function
I	Olfactory	Smell
II	Optic	Vision
III	Oculomotor	Innervation of muscles to move the eyeball, the pupil, and the upper lid
IV	Trochlear	Innervation of superior oblique muscle of eye
V	Trigeminal	Chewing and sensation to face
VI	Abducens	Abducts eye
VII	Facial	Movements of facial muscles, taste, salivary glands
VIII	Vestibular acoustic	Equilibrium and hearing
IX	Glossopharyngeal	Taste, elevation of palate and larynx, salivary glands
X	Vagus	Taste, swallowing, elevation of palate, phonation, parasympathetic outflow to visceral organs
XI	Spinal-accessory	Turning of head and shrugging of shoulders
XII	Hypoglossal	Movement of tongue

sion. Bilateral LMN lesions in children cause severe flaccid dysarthrias, often accompanied by infantile dysphagia (swallowing disorder).

CLINICAL NEUROLOGY OF THE CHILDHOOD DYSARTHRIAS

Upper Motor Neuron Lesions: Spasticity

The clinical concepts of UMN and LMN disorders are particularly helpful in neurologic medicine as well as in speech-language pathology. The understanding of the clinical signs associated with each of these disorders allows the speech-language pathologist to appreciate more clearly the neurologic condition of the child who presents a dysarthria. UMN and LMN syndromes contrast dramatically in the neurologic signs that characterize each of them. The main features that distinguish the two syndromes are based on the type of paralysis, muscle tone, and reflex reactions. These differences are most obvious in the limbs and trunk.

The UMN syndrome is characterized by hyperactive reflexes (hyperreflexia), spasticity, and increased muscle tone (hypertonia). Gilman and

Newman (1987) point out that muscles that display signs of hyperreflexia are said to show spasticity. Spasticity is marked by increased resistance to passive movement of the flexor muscles of the arm and the extensor muscles of the leg. As the physician manipulates the limbs of the child with spasticity through a full range of motion, strong resistance to movement is found at the beginning of the range of movement, but soon the resistance gives way in clasp-knife fashion to less resistance at the end of the range of movement. Although hypertonia may be present in other motor disorders (dystonia, rigidity, myotonia), **clasp-knife spasticity** is typical of spastic hypertonia. Other hypertonic conditions may be differentiated from spasticity in a child by their specific associated distinguishing and confirmatory features.

Confirmatory Signs. Three confirmatory signs are often present in children with spasticity and hyperflexia. They are clonus, spastic weakness of muscles, and the appearance of the Babinski sign. Hyperactive muscle stretch reflexes are expressed in a **clonus**, which is a rapid succession of muscular contraction and relaxation. The presence or absence of ankle clonus is often tested in a spastic child. Clonic movement is characterized by a series of sustained muscle jerks, as when a tendon is maintained in extension by an examining physician. Clonic movements of a dysarthric child's jaw, for instance, may occur spontaneously when the tendon of the jaw musculature is placed under abnormal stretch by environmental stimuli, as sometimes occurs in children with spasticity.

 Spastic muscle weakness, defined as reduced force and muscle velocity, is well documented in the UMN syndrome (Landau, 1974; Travis, 1955). It is present in the muscles of the limbs and digits as well as in the muscles of the oral mechanism (Barlow & Abbs, 1984).

 The **Babinski sign,** a common adult abnormal reflex that appears when the extensor plantar reflex is stimulated, is considered a very stable sign of dysfunction of the corticospinal tract. It is not found in neurologically intact individuals. The sign is elicited by stroking with a blunt object the plantar surface of the outer border of the foot. The normal response is a withdrawal of the foot and a plantar flexion of the great toe—a curling under of the great toe. This plantar flexion of the great toe is sometimes accompanied by a curling under of the other toes. When the Babinski sign is present there is an opposite reaction, a slow dorsiflexion or upward turning of the great toe occasionally accompanied by a fanning of the other toes.

 Although a mainstay in determining corticospinal tract damage in the adult, the Babinski sign is not as reliable a sign of UMN damage in infants and children. In normal infants, a Babinski sign will sometimes appear even though there is no evidence of corticospinal tract damage. The explanation for this paradoxical behavior is based on the fact that the immature nervous system and the damaged nervous system often display similar

TABLE 2-3   Signs of Upper and Lower Motor Neuron Disorder

UMN	LMN
Spastic paralysis	Flaccid paralysis
Hypertonia	Hypotonia
Hyperreflexia	Hyporeflexia
Clonus	No clonus
Babinski sign	No Babinski sign
Little or no atrophy	Marked atrophy
No fasciculations	Fasciculations
Diminished abdominal	Normal abdominal
and cremasteric reflexes	and cremasteric reflexes

signs. Damage to the nervous system will release primitive reflex behavior that has been held in check by higher centers before the damage. The same behavior is seen in the immature nervous system because higher center control has not developed to inhibit primitive reflex behavior. In some children with spasticity, the Babinski sign is a stable sign of brain damage by 2 years of age, but in other children it may not be diagnostic until 10 years. Other reflex signs help to define the UMN syndrome in children, but they will not be discussed here. Table 2-3 presents a comparison of UMN and LMN signs.

Lower Motor Neuron Lesions: Flaccidity

LMN lesions are associated with a variety of etiologies and a wide spectrum of diseases in children. Children with LMN lesions often show similar clinical neurologic signs and present similar dysarthrias even though the etiologies and diseases are diverse. Recall that these varied LMN disorders can be best understood by appreciating that lesions may be at different sites in the motor unit and still present the same typical LMN signs. Comprehensive coverage of the pediatric conditions presenting LMN signs, as well as their associated dysarthrias, is found in Chapter 4.

LMN lesions of the motor neurons in the brain stem, the spinal cord, cranial nerves, or spinal nerves will reduce or abolish normal voluntary movement as well as reflexive activity of the muscles. The resultant paralysis is accompanied by reduced muscle tone, called **hypotonia,** and absence of muscle stretch reflexes, or **areflexia.** The muscle is generally weak, doughy, and flaccid. Usually within a few weeks the muscle begins to **atrophy,** or show a wasting of muscle fibers and a loss of muscle bulk. This atrophy, called **LMN atrophy,** is more severe than is the disuse atrophy that occurs when a muscle has not been used for a period of time.

In the early stages of LMN atrophy, the muscles, including those of the head and neck, may display fibrillations and fasciculations. **Fibrillations** are fine muscle twitchings of single muscle fibers. Although these twitches are not visible to the naked eye, they can be detected with electromyographic (EMG) examination. In contrast, **fasciculations** are described as brief contractions of the motor unit that can be seen just below the skin (Gilman & Newman, 1987). Speech-language pathologists find themselves in a special position to observe fasciculations in LMN disorders because neurologists assert that the muscles of the tongue are one of the most appropriate sites to observe them, since this organ is composed entirely of muscle. In fact, in some LMN diseases the tongue may be shrunken with atrophy and also display fasciculations. Fasciculations have no direct influence on speech production but serve as confirmatory evidence of LMN disease.

Basal Ganglia Lesions: Dyskinesia

Movement disorders in children are generally classified as **dyskinetic** (excessive movement) rather than **akinetic** (lack of movement). Speech-languages pathologists are often familiar with involuntary movement disorders since they usually appear as a subclass of cerebral palsy, the most common neurologic crippling disorder of childhood. One must keep in mind, however, that several specific childhood involuntary movement syndromes other than those in cerebral palsy are marked by dyskinesia and dysarthria. Some of the more common ones include drug-induced tardive dyskinesia, dystonia musculorum deformans, Wilson's disease (hepatolenticular degeneration), and Tourette's syndrome (Fenichel, 1997).

Athetoid cerebral palsy is probably the most common dyskinesia with dysarthria seen in children. **Athetosis** is a slow, writhing movement of the limbs and trunk that may occur alone or in association with chorea, when it is called **choreoathetosis. Chorea** is an involuntary movement disorder characterized by a rapid, fidgety jerk affecting any part of the body. The involuntary movements can be incorporated into a voluntary movement, giving the appearance of restlessness.

Isolated athetosis in children is most commonly caused by hypoxia in the perinatal period, while isolated chorea is seen most often in drug-induced disorders (tardive dyskinesia), systemic disorders, and brain tumor. Choreoathetosis is seen in cerebral palsy, as well as in genetic disorders, infectious diseases, metabolic encephalopathies, and vascular disorders (Fenichel, 1997).

A third major dyskinesia is **dystonia,** which is marked by movements that are slower and more sustained than in chorea or athetosis. The movements distort the affected body part (face, neck, trunk, limbs) into distorted and characteristic dystonic postures that are caused by a simultaneous contraction of agonist and antagonist muscles (Weiner & Lang, 1989). There may be involvement of a single body part (focal dystonia), a limb and contiguous part of the trunk (segmental dystonia), arm and leg on one side (hemidystonia), or involvement of limbs and face (generalized dystonia). If there is a focus in the face and tongue area, the dysarthria (oral-facial dystonic dysarthria) is usually severe.

A genetically transmitted dystonia, called **dystonia musculorum deformans** or primary torsion dystonia, is caused by several forms of dominant and recessive inheritance and usually has an onset between 6 and 14 years. Most cases in childhood start with leg involvement (Marsden & Harrison, 1974). Dystonia, despite the focal feature at onset, always becomes generalized in children so that all four limbs and trunk are involved. In addition to dyskinetic dysarthria, dysphagia and postural tremor are frequent clinical features.

Tardive dyskinesia is another movement disorder syndrome that has a major dysarthric component. In this syndrome, the term dyskinesia is used to describe drug-induced choreiform movements that are limited to the lingual-facial-buccal area. Tardive dyskinesia is caused by the use of drugs, such as the phenothiazines or haloperidol, prescribed to modify behavior in emotional disorders. The incidence is estimated at 1% of the pediatric population (Silverstein & Johnston, 1985). The symptoms include tongue protrusion and lip smacking, which interfere with speech production. Other involuntary movements may occur in the trunk and limbs. In children, the movements usually cease when the drug is discontinued, although this may not be the case in adults.

Other dyskinetic movements such as **tremors** (oscillating movements with a fixed frequency) and **myoclonus** (involuntary movements marked by rapid muscle jerks) rarely play a part in children's speech disorders but have been reported in adult dysarthrias (Darley et al., 1975).

Cerebellum and Cerebellar Pathway Lesions: Ataxia

Ataxia in children results from involvement of the cerebellum and cerebellar pathways. It is considered a disturbance of coordination rather than strength, and the primary sign in children is a wide-based, lurching, staggering gait.

Ataxia may be a major symptom in many pediatric conditions. Acute attacks of ataxia, recurrent attacks of ataxia, and progressive ataxia are often separated from congenital ataxia in children, which is usually chronic and nonprogressive (Fenichel, 1997). Congenital ataxia is considered a major subclass of cerebral palsy along with spasticity and athetosis, although ataxia is the least frequent category of cerebral palsy. Hardy (1983) observes that in the small number of ataxic cerebral-palsied children he has seen, hypotonia and intention or action tremor—tremor associated with an intended movement—are less common than they are in adults. Hypotonia is usually at a peak in neonatal periods and early infancy, and muscle tone increases with age. Congenital ataxic cerebral palsy usually results from malformations of the cerebellum and its pathways or from a genetic disorder. Acquired ataxic cerebral palsy, occurring postnatally, may be caused by cerebellar tumors, infections, trauma, or vascular disorders (Fenichel, 1997; Ingram, 1966). Damage to the left cerebellar hemisphere in either congenital or acquired ataxia is likely to be associated with an ataxic dysarthria (Lectenberg & Gilman, 1978).

CLINICAL NEUROLOGY OF DEVELOPMENTAL VERBAL DYSPRAXIA

Evidence of Brain Dysfunction

One of the several controversial aspects of DVD concerns the nature of the evidence suggesting that it is a true neurologic disorder. Probably the first question that can be raised is this: Is DVD a convincing neurologic analogue of verbal dyspraxia in adults? In the adult brain, the apraxic lesion is most often localized to Broca's convulsion (Area 44) in the left hemisphere. As noted earlier, dyspraxic symptoms also may occur with lesions in the posterior perisylvian area.

The first major study to present neurologic evidence in DVD children was reported by Rosenbek and Wertz (1972). They studied 50 children, identified as having DVD, from retrospective data. Twenty-six children in the sample were examined with electroencephalograms (EEGs). Only 15 of the 26 showed abnormal EEGS. No definite localization of abnormality to the left frontal hemisphere was found. Fourteen of the 50 children demonstrated neurologic signs beyond their dyspraxic speech. Oral apraxia plus other neurologic signs were reported, as well as muscle weakness, spastic muscles, abnormal reflexes, and hyperactive motor patterns.

In a well-known and well-designed study, Yoss and Darley (1974) reported that 15 of the 16 subjects in their clinical apraxic group showed abnormal neurologic findings in terms of "soft" neurologic signs, which are isolated and inconsistent minor neurologic signs. The authors interpreted these signs as pointing to developmental immaturity of the nervous system rather than to actual neurologic dysfunction in terms of a diagnosis of minimal cerebral dysfunction. No objective neurodiagnostic testing was included in this study.

In a careful replication of the Yoss and Darley study, Williams, Ingham, and Rosenthal (1981) found only limited evidence of soft signs in their clinical group and were not able to confirm the pattern of phonologic and prosodic features that Yoss and Darley found in their suspected DVD children. Although the authors did not, in the main, support a concept of developmental apraxia of speech, they did suggest that there might be a subgroup of children, defined by the presence of soft signs, who were indeed speech dyspraxic.

The practice of making the presence of soft signs critical for diagnosis of DVD is hazardous (Love & Fitzgerald, 1984), and it is equally hazardous to assume that soft signs predict cerebral dysfunction in children. The validity and reliability of these signs have been seriously questioned (Kalverboer, van Praag, & Mendlewicz, 1978; Rie & Rie, 1980; Tupper, 1987). At best, minor signs suggest neurologic immaturity, not abnormalities, since such signs often reverse themselves with growth and maturity (Tupper, 1987).

Ferry, Hall, and Hicks (1975) reported on a series of 60 verbal dyspraxics 4 to 30 years of age in which the majority of children (42) were between the ages of 4 and 10 years. This study, which reported EEG findings of mild and nonspecific abnormalities on some of the children in the sample, was also noteworthy for reporting both minor and more obvious neurologic signs in the verbal apraxics. There were 36 instances of orofacial apraxia, 2 cases of mild spastic diplegia, 10 cases of mild motor retardation, 2 instances of hand tremor, and 1 instance each of hemiplegia and choreiform movements. No abnormal gag, pharyngeal, or jaw reflexes were present. There was an absence of lingual atrophy. Interestingly, of those reviewed so far, only this study suggests that some children had actual hard signs of possible neurologic dysfunction.

The most definitive study to date of possible neurologic lesion was reported by Horwitz (1984), who studied 10 children between the ages of 3 and 12 years, with an average age of 7 years, who were diagnosed as verbal apraxics. Diagnostic procedures included computerized tomography (CT) scans, EEGs, and medical laboratory tests deemed necessary in individual patients. The CT scans revealed no consistent gross anatomic basis for the DVD. Seven of the nine scans available were normal. The abnormal scans were dissimilar, one showing enlarged cisterns around the cerebellum and brain stem; the other revealing enlarged occipital borns. Hypotonia was present in the first child, and the second had a medical history of failure to thrive. Normal EEGs and amino acid profiles were typical of the group.

In conclusion, it is clear from the five studies reviewed here that consistent neurologic findings or a specific localized basis has yet to be established for the clinical manifestation of developmental verbal dyspraxia.

SUMMARY

The sections of the motor system involved in speech performance include the cortical level of motor control involving primary motor area (Area 4), the premotor area (lateral Areas 6 and 8) and the supplementary motor area (medial Area 6). Area 44 is a motor planning and programming area for speech and is known as Broca's area, but as yet neurologic research has not associated Broca's area with DVD or developmental oral apraxia in children.

Descending motor pathways from various cortical motor areas provide specific motor control for the body and the speech musculature. The direct motor system includes the corticospinal and corticobulbar tracts. The corticospinal tract is known as the voluntary motor pathway particularly controlling fine movement in the digits and extremities. The corticobulbar tract descends from the motor cortices with the corticospinal tract. It discussates at various levels of the brain stem and ends in the motor neurons of the brain stem, which synapse with the cranial motor nerves for speech (V, VII, IX, X, XI, XII). Lesions to the corticospinal and corticobulbar tracts in children produce a UMN syndrome which is characterized by hypertonia, clasp-knife spasticity, and hyperreflexia in the limbs. There may be an associated spastic dysarthria when corticobulbar tracts are involved.

The indirect motor system includes the basal ganglia and its pathways and the cerebellum and its connections. Both of these structures and their connections influence the direct motor system to provide efficient motor control for movement. Lesions of the basal ganglia and its pathways produce dyskinetic movement disorders of various types. These include chorea, choreoathetosis, athetosis, and dystonia as major disorders in children. Each of these involuntary movement disorders may contribute to dyskinetic dysarthria of childhood with its own features. Common childhood dyskinetic syndromes associated with dysarthria are athetosis of cerebral palsy, tardive dyskinesia (chorea), and dystonia musculorum deformans of childhood. Damage to the cerebellum produces ataxia, which is most commonly seen by the speech-language pathologists as a congenital ataxia of cerebral palsy. It may be accompanied by an ataxic dysarthria.

Damage to the peripheral motor system pathways produces an LMN syndrome. This syndrome may occur with lesions at the various sites in the motor unit. LMN signs include a flaccid muscle paralysis, diminished motor stretch reflexes, atrophy of muscles, and possible fasciculations. The associated childhood dysarthria is a flaccid dysarthria.

SUGGESTED READING

Chusid, J. (1985). *Correlative neuroanatomy and functional neurology* (17th ed.). Los Altos, CA: Lange Medical Publications.

This is a standard basic handbook for students interested in the nervous system. The illustrations are excellent.

Gilman, S., & Newman, S. W. (1987). *Manter and Gatz's essentials of clinical neuroanatomy and neurophysiology* (7th ed.). Philadelphia: F. A. Davis.

A succinct and well-illustrated introduction to the nervous system.

Love, R. J., & Webb, W. G. (1996). *Neurology for the speech-language pathologist* (3rd ed.). Stoneham, MA: Butterworth.

This book provides greater detail on many of the topics considered in this chapter. Chapter 12 deals specifically with issues that relate to childhood motor speech disability.

REFERENCES

Barlow, S. M., & Abbs, J. H. (1984). Orofacial fine-motor control impairments in congenital spasticity: Evidence against hypertonus-related performance deficits. *Neurology, 34,* 145–150.
Barlow, S., & Farley, G. R. (1989). Neurophysiology of speech. In D. P. Kuehn, M. L. Lemme, & J. M. Baumgartner (Eds.), *Neural bases of speech, hearing and language* (pp. 146–200). Boston: Little, Brown.
Brodal, A. (1981). *Neurological anatomy in relation to clinical medicine* (3rd ed.). New York: Oxford University Press.
Bunger, P. (1989). Developmental neuroanatomy and neurophysiology. In D. P. Kuehn, M. L. Lemme, & J. P. Baumgartner (Eds.), *Neural bases of speech, hearing and language* (pp. 87–110). Boston: Little, Brown.
Darley, F. L., Aronson, A., & Brown, J. R. (1975). *Motor speech disorders.* Philadelphia: W. B. Saunders.
Fenichel, G. M. (1997). *Clinical pediatric neurology* (3rd ed.). Philadelphia: W. B. Saunders.
Ferry, P. C., Hall, S. M., & Hicks, J. L. (1975). 'Dilapidated' speech: Developmental verbal apraxia. *Developmental Medicine and Child Neurology, 17,* 749–756.
Gilman, S., & Newman, S. W. (1987). *Manter and Gatz's clinical neuroanatomy and neurophysiology* (7th ed.). Philadelphia: F. A. Davis.
Hardy, J. C. (1983). *Cerebral palsy.* Englewood Cliffs, NJ: Prentice-Hall.
Horwitz, S. J. (1984). Neurological findings in developmental verbal apraxia. *Seminars in Speech and Language, 5,* 111–118.
Ingram, T. T. S. (1966). The neurology of cerebral palsy. *Archives of the Diseases of Children, 41,* 337–357.
Ingvar, D. (1983). Serial aspects of language and speech related to prefrontal cortical activity. *Human Neurobiology, 2,* 177–189.
Kalverboer, A. F., van Praag, H. M., & Mendlewicz, J. (Eds.). (1978). *Minimal brain dysfunction: Fact or fiction.* Basel: Karger.
Kent, R., & Netsell, R. (1978). Articulatory abnormalities in athetoid cerebral palsy. *Journal of Speech and Hearing Disorders, 43,* 353–373.
Landau, W. M. (1974). Spasticity: The fable of a neurological demon and the emperor's new therapy. *Archives of Neurology, 31,* 217–219.
Lectenberg, R., & Gilman, S. (1978). Speech disorders in cerebellar disease. *Annals of Neurology, 3,* 285–289.
Love, R. J., & Fitzgerald, M. (1984). Is the diagnosis of developmental apraxia of speech valid? *Australian Journal of Human Communication Disorders, 12,* 170–178.
Marsden, C. D. (1982). The mysterious motor function of the basal ganglia: The Robert Wartenberg lecture. *Neurology, 32,* 514–539.

Marsden, C. D., & Harrison, M. (1974). Idiopathic torsion dystonia (dystonia musculorum deformans): A review of 42 patients. *Brain, 97,* 793–810.

Mateer, C. A., & Kimura, D. (1977). Impairment of nonverbal oral movements in aphasia. *Brain and Language, 4,* 262–276.

McClean, M. D. (1988). Neuromotor aspects of speech production and dysarthria. In K. M. Yorkston, D. R. Beukelman, & K. R. Bell (Eds.), *Clinical management of dysarthric speakers* (pp. 19–58). Boston: Little, Brown.

Rie, H. D., & Rie, E. D. (1980). *Handbook of minimal brain dysfunctions: A critical view.* New York: John Wiley.

Rosenbek, J., & Wertz, R. (1972). A review of 50 cases of developmental apraxia of speech. *Language, Speech, and Hearing Services in Schools, 3,* 23–33.

Silverstein, F., & Johnston, M. V. (1985). Risks of neuroleptic drugs in children with neurologic disorders. *Annals of Neurology, 18,* 392–397.

Travis, A. M. (1955). Neurological deficits after ablations of the precentral motor area in *Macaca mulatta. Brain, 78,* 155–173.

Tupper, D. E. (Ed.). (1987). *Soft neurological signs.* Orlando, FL: Grune & Stratton.

Weiner, W. J., & Lang, A. E. (1989). *Movement disorders: A comprehensive survey.* Mount Kisco, NY: Futura.

Williams, R., Ingham, R. J., & Rosenthal, R. (1981). A further analysis for developmental apraxia of speech in children with defective articulation. *Journal of Speech and Hearing Research, 24,* 496–505.

Yoss, K. A., & Darley, F. L. (1974). Developmental apraxia of speech in children with defective articulation. *Journal of Speech and Hearing Research, 17,* 339–416.

► **3**

The Childhood Dysarthrias of Cerebral Palsy

In no other clinical population is one likely to find such a va-
riety of conditions that can disturb and delay the acquisition
of oral language as in the group diagnosed as cerebral palsy.
—HAROLD WESTLAKE AND
DAVID RUTHERFORD, 1961

Introduction
    Classification of Dysarthria in Cerebral Palsy

Spastic Syndromes
    Spastic Hemiplegia • Spastic Paraplegia • Spastic Diplegia • Spastic
    Quadriplegia • Speech Mechanism Impairment in Spastic Syndromes •
    Speech Performance in Childhood Spastic Dysarthria

Dyskinetic Syndromes
    Athetoid Syndrome in Cerebral Palsy • Speech Mechanism Impairment
    in Athetosis • Causes of Athetoid Dysarthria

Ataxic Syndromes
    Speech Mechanism Impairment in Ataxic Dysarthria

INTRODUCTION

Cerebral palsy is defined as a nonprogressive disorder of motion and posture due to brain insult or injury occurring in the period of early brain growth, generally under three years of age (Lord, 1984). With an estimated average incidence of two cases per 1000 live births and a prevalence of about 400,000 living children, cerebral palsy is the most common childhood handicapping condition in the United States despite apparent declining incidences (Kudrjacev, Schoenberg, Kurland, & Groover, 1983).

Although the precise prevalence of dysarthria in cerebral palsy is unknown, it is a very frequent sequela of the neurologic disorder. Estimates of the incidence of dysarthria range from 31 to 88% in the early studies of speech disorders in cerebral palsy (Yorkston, Beukelman, & Bell, 1988). Cerebral palsy has many other important sequelae in addition to dysarthria. In fact, cerebral palsy has been called the perfect medical model for demonstrating the wide spectrum of neurologic dysfunctions found in children with developmental disabilities (Denhoff, 1976). Any or all of these additional dysfunctions may compound the developmental dysarthria and/or interfere with communicative performance of the child with cerebral palsy. These dysfunctions include disturbances in cognition, perception, sensation, language, hearing, emotional behavior, feeding, and seizure control.

Classification of Dysarthria in Cerebral Palsy

As indicated in Chapter 2, three major types of dysarthria are generally recognized in cerebral palsy: (1) spastic, (2) dyskinetic, and (3) ataxic. Although no universal classification systems of the clinical types of cerebral palsy exist, many experts currently accept the same major categories of cerebral palsy: spasticity, athetosis (dyskinesia), and ataxia. Each of these three categories may be characterized by different predominating patterns of motor involvement. However, mixtures of abnormal tone and movement disturbances are not uncommon in cerebral-palsied children. (For a discussion of the historical evolution of classification systems in cerebral palsy and attempts to deal with mixed types, see Hardy, 1983, pp. 11–31.)

It should be made clear at this point that over the years, physicians have voiced some discontent with the term *cerebral palsy* as a useful medical diagnosis. The term does not designate a disease in the usual medical sense since there is no single cause, no consistent set of signs and symptoms for all individuals included in the diagnostic category, and no characteristic course (Crothers & Paine, 1959). The designation is only useful in an administrative sense to identify children disabled by motor impairments caused by nonprogressive abnormalities of the brain. Traditionally, the designation of cerebral palsy has emphasized childhood motor impairments that occur in prenatal and perinatal conditions, not those associated with postnatal conditions. Many postnatal conditions resulting in motor disability and dysarthria, such as those caused by meningitides, encephalitides, brain tumors, abscesses, strokes, or other encephalopathies such as Reye's syndrome and pediatric head injury, are described as specific individual syndromes. Similarly, it is helpful to understand the childhood dysarthrias of cerebral palsy by considering them as specific syndromes, even though they may be similar, rather than viewing them as a whole and talking of "cerebral-palsied speech."

SPASTIC SYNDROMES

Spastic syndromes are overwhelmingly the most common type of motor disorder in cerebral palsy in the United States as well as in other countries (Kudrjavcev et al., 1983; Pharaoh, Cooke, Rosenbloom, & Cooke, 1987). Spasticity is often associated with low-birth-weight neonates (under 2500 grams) who experience hypoxia (reduced oxygen) and ischemia (reduced cerebral blood flow), producing **hypoxic-ischemic encephalopathy.** Lesions in these premature infants are frequently in the deep white matter around the ventricles of the brain (Fenichel, 1983). In preterm infants the most common types of cerebral disorder are **periventricular-intraventricular hemorrhage** and **periventricular leukomalacia** resulting from hypoxic-ischemic disorders (DeReuck & Vander Eecken, 1983). This hypoxic-vascular lesion results in four classic types of spastic involvement, each with a predictable clinical picture in relation to speech symptoms.

Spastic Hemiplegia

In the child with **congenital spastic hemiplegia,** the arm and leg on one side of the body show signs of clasp-knife spastic paresis. The corticospinal tract is affected, and the corticobulbar fibers may or may not show involvement. If the corticobulbar fibers are affected, little or no paralysis will occur in the lower half of the face, but there may be involvement of other oral musculature contralateral to the lesion (Lenn & Freinkel, 1989). A prominent cranial nerve sign is hypoglossal (XII) nerve involvement with deviation of the tongue to the side of the body opposite the cerebral lesion. If a dysarthria is present in hemiplegia, the bilateral control of the speech musculature usually allows rapid resolution of what dysarthric elements may be present. Dysphagia may not be a significant problem at all, and if present, it usually reverses itself in a brief period of time.

In the child with a congenital hemiplegia, there may be speech retardation, that is, a mild phonologic delay, sometimes accompanied by language and cognitive disturbances. Early left-hemisphere lesions in children with right hemiplegia appear to be followed by a shift of language centers to the right hemisphere, and language functions survive even after major damage of the hemisphere; but this shift apparently takes a toll in right-hemisphere visual-spatial functions. In children with left hemiplegia and right-hemisphere lesions, language is generally not impaired, but classic signs of right-hemisphere damage in terms of visual-spatial and other functions are present (Woods & Teuber, 1973). In lesions occurring before one year of age, Woods (1987) found that right-hemisphere insult impaired both verbal and performance intelligence quotients. Further, Riva and Cazzaniga (1986) found that lesions occurring before one year produced more severe cognitive impairments than did those occurring after one year of age.

Spastic Paraplegia

In children with **spastic paraplegia**—an uncommon subclass of cerebral palsy—there is involvement of the legs only. Hardy (1983) notes that on occasion muscle involvement may extend into the muscles of the trunk, but the upper extremities are always spared. Even if the respiratory muscles of the trunk become involved to a degree, significant problems are not usually found in speech production. Speech generally develops normally, and significant cognitive impairments are not likely.

Spastic Diplegia

Spastic diplegia implies motor involvement of all four extremities, but the lower limbs show more involvement than do the upper limbs. Sometimes one of the upper limbs shows no involvement and **spastic triplegia** is the result. Respiratory muscles may be affected in addition to the limbs and hands.

The range of dysarthria severity in spastic diplegia is wide. Some children may have a mild disorder involving articulation only, while others may show a more severe problem involving respiratory, laryngeal, articulatory, and palatopharyngeal muscles. Some degree of dysphagia and drooling may be present. Cognitive impairment is found in some cases, but others are intellectually normal.

There is usually flexion and adduction of the hips in the child with diplegia, and "scissoring," or crossing of the legs during walking, produces a classic "scissors gait," a widely known clinical sign of child spasticity. The hamstring muscles of the calf of the leg and the Achilles tendon of the ankle are tight, producing a "toe walker.' In the early literature of cerebral palsy, the spastic diplegic child bore the name "Little's disease" because the first clinical medical description of a diplegic child was that published by William Little (1861).

Spastic Quadriplegia

The child with **spastic quadriplegia** (tetraplegia) displays approximately equal motor involvement in all four limbs, which is generally considered to be the most severe of the spastic syndromes. Usually, the speech musculature is also seriously involved, suggesting that both corticospinal and corticobulbar fibers are compromised in this type of spasticity. Usually respiratory, laryngeal, articulatory, and palatopharyngeal muscles are involved to a noticeable degree, but some children display milder involvement, primarily limited to the oral articulatory muscles (Hardy, 1983). Dysphagia, drooling, and lower facial paralysis with sensory loss of the lips and chin may be present in more severely disabled children. Generally, children with spastic quadriplegia are likely to have a significant degree of cognitive impairment and speech and language delay, although some may be intellectually intact. Mental retardation is usually greater than that found in spastic hemiplegics, paraplegics, or diplegics.

Speech Mechanism Impairment in Spastic Syndromes

Critical motor impairment of the speech mechanism commonly occurs in childhood spastic syndromes in which there is bilateral involvement of the corticobulbar system, namely in those children with diplegia or quadriplegia. As Darley, Aronson, and Brown (1975) point out, four major abnormalities of voluntary movement appear in spastic syndromes with UMN lesions: (1) spasticity, (2) weakness, (3) limitation of range, and (4) slowness of movement. It has been the assumption that in individuals with spasticity, these four abnormalities of motor function similarly disturb movements of the arms and hands as well as movements of the speech mechanism.

Since the classic Mayo Clinic studies of the adult dysarthrias, a series of research reports by various speech scientists have attempted to provide evidence as to whether spastic responses are the same in the muscles of the arms and fingers as they are in the oral muscles of individuals with congenital UMN syndromes. In a significant study, Neilson, Andrews, Guitar, and Quinn (1979) found no evidence of tonic stretch reflex responses in the lip and tongue muscles of congenital spastic subjects with dysarthria. Clearcut tonic stretch reflexes were only associated with the jaw closing muscles, not with jaw opening muscles. From these findings, Neilson and his colleagues concluded that spastic dysarthria could not be attributed to a spastic hypertonus of the lip and tongue muscles presumably caused by hypersensitivity of the tonic stretch reflex. A later study by Barlow and Abbs (1984) of six congenital spastic adults confirmed that hyperactive muscle-spindle based stretch reflexes were apparently not the basis of voluntary orofacial motor impairments in congenital UMN disorder. In this study, the spastic subjects were required to maintain stable muscle force with lips, tongue, and jaw while completing movement tasks with these articulators. Results suggested that control of orofacial fine force was poorer in subjects with spasticity than it was in subjects without spasticity but was not disproportionately poorer in speech muscles like the lips and jaw, which were relatively dense in muscle-spindle innervation. In fact, impairment of the tongue, a muscle system with limited muscle spindles, was more severe than was lip and jaw muscle impairment. Poor orofacial motor performance was characterized by slow and variable movement trajectories in the experimental tasks. Instability of fine-force control of the articulators was highly correlated with instrumental measures of speech performance such as air flow measures in the speech mechanism. In summary, it appeared that orofacial movement and force abilities in spasticity are marked by muscle weakness and instability of force that are unrelated to any spastic hypertonus in the speech muscles.

A further report on congenital spastic adults by Barlow and Abbs (1986) indicated that despite articulator weakness and movement velocity deficits, spastic subjects were able to reach endpoint targets accurately in terms of both muscle force and position. The average movement velocities and average rate in change of force were significantly correlated with a widely used clinical measurement of intelligibility of speech called *Assessment of Intelligibility of Dysarthric Speech* (Yorkston & Beukelman, 1981). Interestingly, mild speech intelligibility impairments on this test, in the 5 to 10% range, were often accompanied by very dramatic reductions in orofacial force control. Moreover, it is apparent that the fine-force and movement impairments were not uniform for the orofacial structures tested. In three of the five subjects, a standard clinical assessment of the oral motor systems and speech indicated normal function, but the physiologic laboratory testing of force and movement revealed significant impairments in the articulator control in spasticity that were not apparent during routine clinical examination. Barlow and Abbs argue that measures such as these may be particularly useful in evaluation results of intervention programs. However, the greatest value of their research probably is in their definition of specific relationships of muscle weakness, articulator instability, and target accuracy in dysarthria in congenital spasticity. Before this significant research, these relationships in the orofacial control problems of spastic dysarthria had not been clarified for the speech-language pathologist.

Speech Performance in Childhood Spastic Dysarthria

Respiratory Function. The child with bilateral spasticity commonly displays abnormalities in quiet and speech breathing. Studies of respiratory function often have combined both spastic and athetoid children and have reported similar problems in both major subgroups of cerebral palsy. Blumberg (1955) studied 13 spastic, 12 athetoid, and 2 ataxic children. The children with spasticity were reported to have milder disturbances of phonation, loudness, and general respiratory control than did children with athetosis. Breathing rates, rhythm, volume, and depth of inhalation were also reported to be more normal in the children with spasticity. Achilles (1955) confirmed this superiority in respiratory control of spastic individuals.

In a later, well-known, carefully executed study of the respiratory function of spastic and athetoid speakers with cerebral palsy, Hardy (1964) reported that spastic quadriplegic children had reduced respiratory reserve and subsequent lowered vital capacities. Reviewing these findings in 1983, Hardy suggested that the reduced ability of the spastic subgroups to expire below their resting respiratory levels was probably due in large part to involvement of their abdominal wall muscles. As we have already noted, this respiratory deficit may even be present in mild spastic paraplegic children as well as in other spastic children. In severely disabling cases of paraplegia and diplegia, reduced expiratory capacity may result from the added involvement of the thoracic wall muscles to the already disturbed abdominal muscles.

The reduction of vital capacity that is common in children with spasticity is not necessarily associated with inadequate breath support for speech, according to Hardy (1983). He believes that there generally is no direct cause-effect relationship between reductions in vital capacity and speech production; it is only when laryngeal, velopharyngeal, or articulatory dysfunctions interact with the respiratory dysfunctions that overall speech function may become clinically impaired. In certain instances, since a spastic child generally utilizes more air volume per syllable than does a normal child, poor valving of the airstream results in limited respiratory support for speech and short phrasing of utterance.

Laryngeal Function.   Dysfunction of the laryngeal muscles has been reported widely among children with cerebral palsy, but few instrumental studies have been devoted to describing the phonatory deficits specific to spastic children. Clinical observations by Ingram (1966) suggest that diplegic children present a characteristic phonatory-prosodic pattern, a "monotony of intonation and stress patterns" (p. 345). This suggests loudness and pitch deviations like those currently described as symptoms of monopitch and monoloudness in adult dysarthria (Darley et al., 1975). In spastic diplegia cases, I personally have observed increased voice onset times, harsh voice, and short phrasing. This last problem no doubt is the result of poor respiratory function plus air wastage at the laryngeal level because of poor valving at the glottis. Occasionally, I have heard the struggle-strangle voice quality reported in adult spastics and intermittent dysphonia, probably due to laryngeal stenosis as a result of hypertonic vocal folds. Laryngeal deviations have not been specifically reported for childhood spastic quadriplegics, but it is my observation that they may generally present more deviant vocal characteristics than do diplegics. Laryngeal involvement may even result in aphonia in some children. Along with the struggle-strangle vocal elements, monopitch and loudness are not uncommon. The lack of instrumental research in this area of childhood spastic dysarthria is critical, since the changing characteristics of the cerebral-palsied population suggest that spastic subgroups will soon be the major concern.

Velopharyngeal Function.   In recent years, disorders of velopharyngeal closure have been highlighted as critical speech deficits in cerebral palsy, although early work tended to discount these disorders (McDonald & Chance, 1964). The seminal work of Netsell (1969) stands out in this regard. Studying a group of cerebral-palsied children including those with spasticity, Netsell recorded intraoral breath pressure, rate of nasal airflow, and several speech-signal characteristics to determine palatopharyngeal competence in cerebral palsy. He found five deviations in palatopharyngeal competence worth noting:

1. gradual opening of the velopharyngeal port during the utterance of a series of syllables;
2. gradual closing of the port when a series of syllables was speeded up;
3. premature opening of the port as a series of syllables was begun;
4. bursts of airflow after a given syllable in an utterance because of the tentative opening of the velopharyngeal port; and
5. breaking of the velopharyngeal seal when nonnasal consonant sounds were produced.

This careful laboratory study clearly supported the assertions of long-time observers of the speech of cerebral-palsied individuals that velopharyngeal problems were of significance in the population. Over a generation ago, Ingram and Barn (1961) reported hypernasality and nasal escapage as common speech problems of spastic diplegic, double hemiplegic, and tetraplegic children in Edinburgh, Scotland. Currently, it is believed that management of velopharyngeal impairments not only resolves resonance problems but also improves articulation and airflow throughout the speech mechanism. The result is a much-improved overall speech performance (Hardy, 1983).

Articulatory Function.   Phonologic development and disorders have been the objects of the most extensive research of any aspect of speech performance in cerebral palsy. The most ambitious research program on various facets of articulation in cerebral palsy was undertaken over a 10-year period by Irwin (1972). He developed a series of standardized articulation tests of various types and lengths to assess vowel and consonant proficiency in terms of manner, place, voicing, and type of articulation, and he tested hundreds of children in several states in the United States. Findings were generally similar for spastic and athetoid children, although the spastic children were typically slightly superior to the athetoid children in terms of scores on Irwin's *Integrated Test of Articulation for Cerebral-Palsied Children*. Differences in error scores and error patterns certainly were not great enough between the two groups for a speech-language pathologist to identify the clinical type of cerebral palsy of a given child by his or her articulation test results, but population trends were clear. Spastic paraplegic children made fewer errors than did hemiplegic children, and hemiplegics made fewer errors than did quadriplegic children. In general, the effect of chronological ages, mental ages, and IQs were negligible on the scores, suggesting that the severity of oromotor involvement was the most critical variable in the dysarthrias of cerebral palsy.

In terms of the manner of articulation for the sample as a whole, labial phonemes were the easiest for the population to produce correctly, and dentals and glottals the most difficult. As for place of articulation, the nasals were the least difficult in the initial and final positions of words, while fricatives and glides were the most difficult in all positions. Voiced consonants were less difficult than were their voiceless cognates. Omission errors tended to exceed substitution of phonemes, a finding that is the reverse of the finding in normal children.

Lencione (1953) and Byrne (1959) contributed two cross-sectional studies of articulation acquisition in cerebral palsy. Byrne reported on spastic and athetoid quadriplegic children between the ages of 2 and 7 years, and Lencione studied a group of similar children 8 to 14 years of age. In her study, Byrne found superior articulation scores for spastics, but these scores were not statistically different, while the difference between the older subgroups was statistically significant in Lencione's study. Articulation development was significantly delayed in the young children studied, but the phoneme acquisition pattern followed a similar course in both normal and cerebral-palsied children. Phoneme proficiency was greatest for bilabials in the young cerebral-palsied child, a finding similar to that of normal children. The more complex tongue-tip and back-of-the-tongue phonemes, which appear later in the speech of normal children, were less often produced correctly in the speech of cerebral-palsied children. Byrne argued from these data that the pattern of articulation acquisition in children with cerebral palsy was determined by the motor complexity of the phoneme to be acquired. Less motor-complex phonemes were easier for a motor-disabled child to produce and were therefore acquired earlier, while more complex sounds were more difficult for the child and appeared later in the schedule of articulation acquisition. Byrne's advocacy of a *motor-complexity principle* for determining phoneme acquisition in child dysarthrias was criticized on the grounds that the principle operated equally in articulation acquisition in normal children, but a more recent study by Platt, Andrews, Young, and Quinn (1980) of articulation skills in adult cerebral-palsied subjects has provided data to support Byrne's contention about the importance of motor complexity.

Hixon and Hardy (1964) studied the severity of articulation defectiveness, rates of syllable diadochokinesis, and nonspeech diadochokinesis in spastic and athetoid children and determined that syllable diadochokinesis was a much better predictor of articulation severity than was nonspeech diadochokinesis. Love, Hagerman, and Tiami (1980) reported that in older cerebral-palsied individuals displaying abnormal oral reflexes, there was no systematic relationship between the number of oral reflexes and articulation proficiency. Platt et al. (1980) and Platt, Andrews, and Howie (1980) reported that articulation patterns of adults with spastic and athetoid cerebral palsy indicated that articulatory error patterns did not distinguish the two subgroups. The rates of speech diadochokinesis in the total sample were 50% slower than that of normal adults. Both spastic and athetoid adult subgroups demonstrated imprecision in fricative and affricative production and had difficulty in achieving extreme articulatory gestures in the articulator space. These subjects, for the most part, produced within manner errors. Errors of place of articulation that crossed expected articulatory boundaries were uncommon. Athetoid speakers, however, made more errors of place than did spastic speakers, suggesting more target inaccuracy of articulation in dyskinetic dysarthria. In summary, the intelligibility of adult cerebral-palsied articulation was poor even after years of speech training and appeared to be related to the severity of oromotor involvement.

Over the years, attempts have been made to determine whether the speech of spastic and athetoid subgroups could be differentiated by listener judgment. The early studies by Rutherford (1944) and Leith and Steer (1958) using judgments of rate, pitch, loudness, articulation, and intelligibility were largely unsuccessful in differentiating between the two subgroups. Platt et al. (1980) reported that the speech of adult spastic speakers was more intelligible and less articulatory-impaired than was the speech of individuals with athetosis. Clarke and Hoops (1980) studied spastic and athetoid children to determine the number of articulation errors, intelligibility, mean fundamental frequency, variation of fundamental frequency, mean sound pressure level, variation in sound pressure level, and the reading rate of words and found spastic subjects tended to be better than athetoid subjects in articulatory ability, intelligibility, and reading rate. Workinger and Kent (1991) reported differences between the two groups but found much overlap in perceptual characteristics of their dysarthrias.

In summary, children with spastic syndromes appear to show less severe speech impairment than do children with an athetoid syndrome. Moreover, predictability of clinical subgroups by listener judgment alone must involve several speech attributes. At present, reliable clinical diagnosis of subtype should include listener judgment in addition to observable neurologic signs.

DYSKINETIC SYNDROMES

Athetosis is the most common dyskinetic syndrome of cerebral palsy. It may appear in a pure form or be the major component in a mixture of dyskinetic symptoms, such as choreoathetosis or dystonic athetosis. In whatever form, its occurrence in the cerebral-palsied population is much less frequent than are spastic syndromes. Erenberg (1984) reports that 5% of the total cerebral-palsied population is pure athetoid and 10% is dystonic athetoid. Pharoah et al. (1987) report only 4% of their sample of 685 children in Liverpool, England, were dyskinetic. Although clinical diagnoses and percentages vary from study to study, there is considerable agreement among experts that the occurrence of the different forms of cerebral palsy is changing dramatically. Over the past half century, the most common type of athetoid cerebral palsy was caused by kernicterus, a condition in which brain injury occurred because of blood-type incompatibilities between a pregnant mother and her unborn child. Rh incompatibility was the most common of the hemolytic incompatibilities. The ability to prevent Rh sensitization has brought about a significant decline in kernicterus and thus in athetoid cerebral palsy (Clarke, 1968). Athetosis, often with signs of choreoathetosis, is now predominantly caused in cerebral palsy by perinatal anoxia. Choreoathetosis may be seen in cerebral palsy, as well as in other childhood neurologic conditions, such as those caused by infections, genetic disorders, and metabolic disturbances (Fenichel, 1997).

Athetoid Syndrome in Cerebral Palsy

Hypotonia and slow motor development are often the first signs of a motor disability in the athetoid child. There is a failure to achieve sitting balance and the well-known infantile reflexes reactions such as the Moro reflex and the asymmetric tonic neck reflex (ATNR) are abnormal (Figures 3-1 and 3-2). As the child matures, the hypotonia may progress to normal tone or a mixed hypertonic-athetoid condition (mixed spastic-athetoid). Generally, there is involvement of all four extremities and the child is commonly diagnosed as an athetoid quadriplegic. Rarely is athetosis limited to less than all four limbs. The speech mechanism is frequently involved. There is often a history of early dysphagia and drooling, and chronic dysphagia and dysarthria are common. Cognitive deficits may or may not accompany the motor disability. In general, the severity of the dyskinetic involvement of the limbs is correlated with the severity of speech mechanism involvement, but several cases have been reported with severe limb involvement and little or no involvement of the speech mechanism. Certainly no perfect correlation exists between the severity of involuntary limb movements and the severity of involvement of the midline speech muscles (Hardy, 1983).

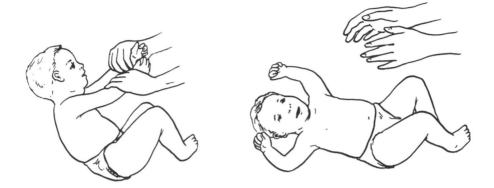

FIGURE 3-1   Moro Reflex
This reflex is elicited by dropping the infant's head or producing a loud
noise. The reflex is pathologic if there is a persistent symmetrical adduction
and upward movement of the arms with fingers splayed, followed by a
flexion of arms in clasp manner.

Source: From *Neurology for the Speech-Language Pathologist* (3rd ed.) by R. J. Love and W. G.
Webb, 1996, Stoneham, MA: Butterworth Publishers. Copyright 1996 by Butterworth
Publishers. Reprinted by permission.

Speech Mechanism Impairment in Athetosis

Respiratory Function.   Athetoid children and adults often show impairments in every major component of the speech mechanism. Respiratory and
laryngeal problems have received considerable attention in the literature.
Respiration in the infant who develops lithetosis is often very rapid and irregular (Davis, 1987). Infantile breathing and phonation is mediated at the
brain stem level with the nuclei in the midbrain and pons responsible for this
function. Grey matter around the aqueduct of the ventricular system, known
as the **periaqueduct area,** is important for integration of phonation at lower
levels of the nervous system. Motor control for the vocal system develops
outward both cephalically and caudally from the brain stem (Stark, 1985).
Cerebral damage of the periaqueduct area is common in hypoxic-ischemic
disorders of neonates who may develop either athetosis or spasticity, according to Fenichel (1997). This damage may delay or disrupt the development of higher neural centers that control respiration in cerebral-palsied
children. The result may be a disturbance in the normal slowing of the
breathing rate that comes with age and a disorder in the regulation of breathing patterns in the athetoid child.

Another aspect of infantile breathing that may persist in the athetoid
child is what has been called **belly breathing.** During the first six months of

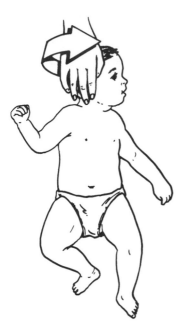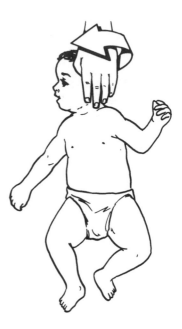

FIGURE 3-2   Asymmetrical Tonic Neck Reflex
This reflex is elicited by turning the infant's head to each side for 5 seconds.
This should be repeated five times to each side. The reflex is pathologic if
there is obligatory extension and flexion of limbs for more than 60 seconds.

Source: From *Neurology for the Speech-Language Pathologist* (3rd ed.) by R. J. Love and W. G.
Webb, 1996, Stoneham, MA: Butterworth Publishers. Copyright 1996 by Butterworth
Publishers. Reprinted by permission.

life, respiratory patterns of normal infants are marked by the greatest movement in the abdominal area during inspiration. Belly breathing is brought
about by contraction of the diaphragm with little or no thoracic expansion.
What little thoracic movement that does occur consists of lowering the floor
of the thoracic cavity. The vertebral column and thorax do not yet provide
adequate support for upper thoracic expansion in the infant (Davis, 1987).
Normal weight-shifting patterns that occur in the 3- to 6-month period of infancy activate and strengthen the thoracic muscles that ultimately will be
used in more mature breathing. Around the 6th month, mid-thoracic excur-
sions can be seen during inspiration. As the child achieves a sitting posture,
there is a normal extension of the vertebral column and thorax against grav-
ity. Rotation patterns of the body develop and elongate the oblique abdominal muscles and the intercostal muscles diagonally. This allows thoracic
movement in three dimensions, and this in turn promotes increased respira-

tory activity (Davis, 1987). In athetoid children, lack of stability and extension of the vertebral column as well as delayed head balance and sitting posture result in breathing patterns of the neonate that persist into later childhood.

Paradoxical or reverse breathing is a typical abnormal pattern of breathing in athetoids (Hardy, 1983; Westlake & Rutherford, 1961). It is identified by a depression of the upper chest during inhalation with a flattening of the sternum and flaring of the lower rib margins. It is usually attributed to a lack of strength of the upper chest and neck muscles to counteract the forceful contraction of the diaphragm. During inspiration these muscles do not fix the rib cage against negative intrathoracic pressure created by the downward movement of the diaphragm. The result is a rib cage of limited size and a reduced volume of air during inhalation. The effect on speech breathing is problematic. Hardy notes that reverse breathing appears more commonly in the athetoid cerebral-palsied child because often there is relatively more severe involvement of the thoracic wall muscles as compared to abdominal wall muscles in these children. Hardy believes that the powerful inspiratory muscle, the diaphragm, is usually spared, providing for a tendency toward flared lower ribs. The reverse breathing pattern, he believes, will reduce the vital capacity to a degree, but will not be a major hazard to speech production in most instances.

Hardy also points out that respiratory dysfunction may contribute to limitations in pitch and loudness due to increased subglottal air pressure. Fundamental frequency is raised with increased subglottal pressure. Further, the often-observed substitution of voiced consonants for their voiceless cognates seems to result from an attempt to conserve respiratory effort. Clearly, respiratory problems have several potentially negative effects on speech performance in dyskinetic dysarthria.

Laryngeal Function. Laryngeal dysfunction is also commonplace in athetoid children. In very early research, Rutherford (1944) observed monotony of pitch in the athetoid speaker. Clement and Twitchell (1959) described the voices of athetoids as low in pitch with weak intensity and a forced voice quality. Hardy (1983) has suggested that in some severely involved athetoid children air rushes through the vocal tract with no phonation occurring. This laryngeal behavior suggests an inability to adduct the vocal folds to the midline of the glottis. Milder laryngeal dysfunction may result in weak vocal intensity and a breathy quality when the vocal folds improperly adduct, resulting in insufficient tension in the folds.

Hyperadduction of the vocal folds, on the other hand, may result in a lack of phonation. Lack of phonation may occur not only as a result of specific hyperadduction of the folds but also as a result of a generalized hypertonic muscle contraction, which immobilizes the whole vocal mechanism.

When the athetoid individual with laryngeal immobilization syndrome does phonate, his or her voice usually has a strained quality with initial audible glottal attack accompanied by an inability to sustain phonation. Vocal fold tension also may be poorly regulated, resulting in a voice marked by a monotone or inappropriate pitch variation (McDonald, 1987).

In brief, limited instrumental research in this area has been reported, and the literature is characterized by the previously mentioned opinions of experts rather than by extensive empirical data, yet laryngeal dysfunction remains a major problem in many cerebral-palsied dysarthrics.

Articulatory Dysfunction.   Kent and Netsell (1978) have provided a cineradiographic report on five athetoid cerebral-palsied subjects 7 through 26 years of age. Vocal tract configurations were studied for the articulation of isolated vowels, VCV nonsense utterances, and short sentences. The most frequent oral articulatory abnormalities were (1) large ranges of jaw movement, (2) inappropriate positioning of the tongue for phonetic segments because of a reduced range of tongue movement, (3) instability of velar elevation, (4) prolonged transition times for articulatory movements, and (5) retrusion of the lower lip.

Explanations for the abnormally large ranges of jaw movements common to all subjects are at best speculative, but it is clear that in athetosis the jaw may act as a much more critical articulator than it does in normal individuals. Tongue movements were largely dependent on jaw movements in this study. In fact, in these subjects jaw movement was the prime mover for tongue movements. Tongue height for isolated articulatory targets and targets in context varied with the ability of athetoids to control their mandibles. The athetoid subjects showed reduction in the anterior-posterior positioning of the tongue, which distorted positions for the vowels. If the jaw is indeed a prime mover in tongue movement, it certainly cannot compensate for the inadequacies of anterior-posterior tongue movement, and phoneme distortion is the result.

The authors further observed that athetoid speakers were unable to perform fine shaping of the tongue for consonant articulation. The limited range of tongue movements and the grossness of tongue shaping appeared to be the causes of abnormally long transition times between articulatory movements.

All subjects had some difficulty in achieving velopharyngeal closure and in maintaining velar position. The velum appeared to move inappropriately, causing velopharyngeal inadequacy during nonnasal sequences. Moreover, the speed of velar movements was slower and more variable than it is in normal individuals. Although the exact reason for these abnormalities in oral articulatory control is unknown, it is quite clear that dyskinetic movements of the oral mechanism are very similar to dyskinetic movements of the extremities of athetoids in that movements show the same type of abnormal motor control. Unlike oral muscle control in spasticity, which apparently is different than limb muscle control, the oral muscle system and the limb muscle system in athetoid dyskinesia seem to display similar disorders of muscle control.

Causes of Athetoid Dysarthria

In two interesting publications, Neilson and O'Dwyer (1981, 1984) have searched for the pathophysiologic mechanisms that might cause dysarthria in cerebral palsy, particularly in the athetoid cerebral-palsied individual. Both the speech and neurologic literature have implied that the dysarthria of athetosis in cerebral palsy is caused by variable, irregular, and even random involuntary movements of the speech muscles. Neilson and O'Dwyer (1984) have questioned this conventional view of the basis of dysarthria in athetosis. Based primarily on electromyographic (EMG) evidence, the researchers have demonstrated that their athetoid subjects were able to successfully repeat the same articulation in the syllables of a test sentence when they were asked to reproduce that sentence. Involuntary activity intermittently occurred in the time intervals between syllables in the sentence but did not occur during the articulation of the syllables themselves. The EMG activity associated with each syllable in the sentence was grossly abnormal in the reproducible or repeatable portion of the EMG recordings. From this data Neilson and O'Dwyer argue that abnormal voluntary activity, rather than variable and random involuntary activity, is the basis for athetoid dysarthria.

Earlier research (1981) on cerebral-palsied adults had allowed Neilson and O'Dwyer to rule out competing theories of the possible cause of dysarthria in cerebral palsy. These theories included:

1. inefficient valving of the airstream caused by paresis of the speech musculature (Hardy, 1964, 1967);
2. abnormalities of tone due to sustained EMG background activity (Netsell, 1975);
3. primitive or pathologic reflexes interfering with articulatory control (Crickmay, 1966; Mysak, 1963);
4. imbalance between positive and negative oral responses (Clement & Twitchell, 1959; Twitchell, 1961); or
5. disruption of voluntary activity usually associated with athetosis (Ingram & Barn, 1961; Paine & Oppe, 1966).

Neilson and O'Dwyer (1984) present data from their research to discount these five theories for the cause of dysarthria in athetoid cerebral palsy and propose that a pattern of abnormal voluntary motor commands for speech is generated by athetoids rather than a set of involuntary movements.

The researchers assume that inappropriate commands arise in athetosis because cerebral lesions preclude normal sensorimotor integration for generating appropriate motor commands for speech. Disruption of the internal sensorimotor feedback system for appropriate motor commands leads to the generation of faulty movements that are perceived by others and by athetoid individuals themselves as involuntary. The clear significance of this study is that systematic research such as this on dyskinetic speech movement problems may clarify underlying neural mechanisms of speech production in certain types of dysarthria that were not readily apparent in the earlier speech and neurologic literature. A summary of common speech symptoms in athetoids and spastics is found in Table 3-1.

ATAXIC SYNDROMES

Ataxia continues to be an uncommon syndrome in cerebral palsy (Crothers & Paine, 1959; Hardy, 1983). Pharoah et al. (1987) report the incidence of ataxia as 4.2% in their sample. Other recent authors do not even mention the classification (Erenberg, 1984). The disorder in ataxic cerebral palsy is primarily one of incoordination (dyssynergia), and the most significant sign in children is a wide-based, lurching, staggering gait (Fenichel, (1997). Other classic signs of the disorder that may be present in ataxic cerebral palsy are hypotonia, dysmetria, action tremor, and nystagmus (see Chapter 2). Etiologies of congenital chronic ataxias include cerebellar malformation, metabolic disturbances, birth trauma, and genetic disorders (Fenichel, 1997; Ingram, 1966). Mixed ataxic-spastic children have been reported as a frequent subtype. These children usually have spastic signs in the lower limbs and are labelled ataxic diplegics (Ingram, 1966).

Speech Mechanism Impairment in Ataxic Dysarthria

Systematic studies of the speech of ataxic dysarthric children have not been reported, but clinical observations suggest that the speech characteristics in ataxic cerebral palsy are very similar to those of the adult with ataxic dysarthria. Ingram lists the following speech signs in ataxic cerebral palsy: speech retardation, inconsistency of substitutions and omissions of sounds, scanning speech, and dysrhythmia and associated disorders of intonation and stress.

Darley et al. (1975) reported 10 deviant perceptual speech dimensions in adult ataxic dysarthria, including imprecise consonants, irregular articulatory breakdown, distorted vowels, excess and equal stress, prolonged

TABLE 3-1 Common Speech Symptoms in the Childhood Dysarthrias of Spastics and Athetoids

Respiration	Phonation	Resonance	Articulation	Prosody
Rapid rate	Poor pitch control	Hypernasality	Spastics slightly superior to athetoids	Reduced variations in intensity, frequency, and timing
Abdominal breathing	Poor loudness control	Nasal emission	Articulation development systematic but delayed	Voice commonly monotone through utterance
Reverse or paradoxical breathing in athetoids	Monotone	Poor intraoral breath pressure	Motor complex sounds more difficult	Slowed rate
Limited upper thorax expansion	Breathiness	Varying types of velopharyngeal inadequacy	Athetoids use wide range of movement of articulators	No formal studies of prosody
Flared lower ribs	Poor adduction/abduction of vocal folds	Inconsistency of velopharyngeal closure	Also uses jaw as major articulator	
Poor tidal air control	Varying tension of vocal folds	Incoordination of velar musculature	Adults show oral motion rates 50% slower than normal	
Increased subglottal pressure	Generalized laryngeal immobility		Athetoids show some out-of-class substitution; spastics do not	
Poor timing of voice and respiration				

phonemes, slow rate monopitch, monoloudness, and harsh voice. They suggested that articulatory inaccuracy was due to errors of individual movements and dysrhythmia of repetitive movements. Prosodic excess was the result of slow individual and repetitive oral movements, and phonatory-prosodic insufficiency was the result of hypotonia. This description of ataxic dysarthria in adults plus further descriptions by Kent and Netsell (1975) and Kent, Netsell, and Abbs (1979) appear similar to Ingram's early clinical descriptions of ataxic dysarthria in cerebral palsy. Two points should be made from personal clinical observations about the speech disorder in ataxic cerebral palsy. First, the severity of articulation disorder may be related more closely to general intellectual levels than to the degree of oromotor disability. Second, ataxic dysarthria in cerebral palsy may present as a generally mild disorder (usually milder than spastic or athetoid dysarthrias); when it does, it may be difficult to separate from general developmental phonological impairment of young children.

SUMMARY

Cerebral palsy is a nonprogressive disorder of motion and posture due to brain insult or injury generally occurring before the age of three years. Three major types of cerebral palsy are widely recognized: spasticity, dyskinesia (predominantly athetosis), and ataxia. Each of these major types is associated with a characteristic dysarthria: spastic, dyskinetic, or ataxic. Spastic syndromes now predominate in the cerebral-palsied population. Four major types are recognized: spastic hemiplegia, paraplegia, diplegia, and quadriplegia. Spastic diplegics and quadriplegics are more likely to have speech disorders. Muscle-spindle based hypertonus does not appear to play a role in speech movement impairment in spastic syndromes; but muscle weakness, articulator instability, and accuracy in finding target articulation points characterize the oral movements of spastic individuals.

Children with spasticity are slightly superior to those with athetosis in respiratory functions and articulatory functions. Serious laryngeal control problems may be present in both spastic and athetoid subgroups, although these laryngeal problems have not yet been systematically studied in the speech laboratory. Velopharyngeal dysfunction is common to both spastic and athetoid groups and appears to be a major hazard to normal resonance, articulation, and intelligibility. The principle of motor complexity to explain articulation acquisition in cerebral palsy is useful for interpreting patterns of articulation errors in adults as well as children. Many adults with cerebral palsy often remain seriously impaired in terms of speech intelligibility and oral-motor movements, despite prolonged efforts at speech training.

Athetoid children represent the most frequent type of childhood dyskinetic dysarthria. The dysarthria appears to be caused by faulty programming of voluntary movements rather than being the result of random involuntary movements.

Congenital ataxic cerebral palsy is uncommon, and little research has been reported concerning its speech characteristics, but clinical evidence points to the fact that it is very similar to the well-described ataxic dysarthria in adults.

Despite a changing incidence of clinical types in cerebral palsy and an apparently declining incidence of cerebral palsy as a whole, the childhood dysarthrias of the cerebral palsies remain the most common childhood motor speech disability in the United States.

SUGGESTED READING

Hardy, J. C. (1983). *Cerebral palsy.* Englewood Cliffs, NJ: Prentice-Hall.

This book, by a well-known speech expert, deals primarily with the developmental dysarthrias of cerebral palsy but also contains insights into several other aspects of cerebral palsy.

Miller, G., & Clark, G. D. (Eds.). (1988). *The cerebral palsies.* Boston: Butterworth-Heinemann.

A recent, comprehensive review of the issues created by cerebral palsy. The approach taken is almost entirely medical.

Stark, R. E. (1985). Dysarthria in children. In J. B. Darby (Ed.), *Speech and language evaluation in neurology: Childhood disorders* (pp. 185–217). New York: Grune & Stratton.

This chapter is a nice blend of information from neurology and speech science brought to bear on the problems of dysarthria of children. The emphasis is on the dysarthrias of cerebral palsy, and evaluation is emphasized.

Thompson, G. H., Rubin, I. L., & Bilenker, R. M. (Eds.). (1983). *Comprehensive management of cerebral palsy.* New York: Grune & Stratton.

This book presents excellent reviews of the disorder and its management. The chapters on the medical aspects of treatment are particularly good.

REFERENCES

Achilles, R. (1955). Communication anomalies of individuals with cerebral palsy. I. Analysis of communication processes in 151 cases of cerebral palsy. *Cerebral Palsy Review, 16,* 15–24.

Barlow, S. M., & Abbs, J. H. (1984). Orofacial fine-motor control impairments in congenital spasticity: Evidence against hypertonus-related performance deficits. *Neurology, 34,* 145–150.

Barlow, S. M., & Abbs, J. H. (1986). Fine force and position control of selected orofacial structures in the upper motor neuron syndrome. *Experimental Neurology, 94,* 699–713.

Blumberg, M. (1955). Respiration and speech in the cerebral palsied child. *American Journal of the Diseases of Children, 89,* 48–53.

Byrne, M. (1959). Speech and language development in athetoid and spastic children. *Journal of Speech and Hearing Disorders, 24,* 231–240.

Clarke, C. A. (1968). The prevention of 'rhesus' babies. *Scientific American, 119* (November), 46–52.

Clarke, W. M., & Hoops, H. R. (1980). Predictive measures of speech proficiency in cerebral palsied speakers. *Journal of Communication Disorders, 13,* 385–394.

Clement, M., & Twitchell, T. E. (1959). Dysarthria in cerebral palsy. *Journal of Speech and Hearing Disorders, 24,* 118–122.

Crickmay, M. C. (1966). *Speech therapy and the Bobath approach to cerebral palsy.* Springfield, IL: C. C. Thomas.

Crothers, B., & Paine, R. (1959). *The natural history of cerebral palsy.* Cambridge, MA: Harvard University Press.

Darley, F. L., Aronson, A. E., & Brown, J. E. (1975). *Motor speech disorders.* Philadelphia: W. B. Saunders.

Davis, L. F. (1987). Respiration and phonation in cerebral palsy. *Seminars in Speech and Language, 8,* 101–106.

Denhoff, E. (1976). Medical aspects. In W. M. Cruickshank (Ed.), *Cerebral palsy: A developmental disability* (3rd rev. ed., pp. 31–71). Syracuse, NY: Syracuse University Press.

De Reuck, J., & Vander Eecken, H. (1983). Brain maturation and types of perinatal hypoxic-ischemic encephalopathy. *European Neurology, 22,* 261–264.

Erenberg, G. (1984). Cerebral palsy. *Postgraduate Medicine, 75,* 87–93.

Fenichel, G. M. (1983). Hypoxic-ischemic encephalopathy in the newborn. *Archives of Neurology, 40,* 261–266.

Fenichel, G. M. (1997). *Clinical pediatric neurology* (3rd ed.). Philadelphia: W. B. Saunders.

Hardy, J. C. (1964). Lung function of athetoid and spastic quadriplegic children. *Developmental Medicine and Child Neurology, 6,* 378–388.

Hardy, J. C. (1967). Suggestions for physiologic research in dysarthria. *Cortex, 3,* 128–156.

Hardy, J. C. (1983). *Cerebral palsy.* Englewood Cliffs, NJ: Prentice-Hall.

Hixon, T. J., & Hardy, J. C. (1964). Restricted motility of the speech articulators in cerebral palsy. *Journal of Speech and Hearing Disorders, 29,* 293–306.

Ingram, T. T. S. (1966). The neurology of cerebral palsy. *Archives of Diseases of Childhood, 41,* 337–357.

Ingram, T. T. S., & Barn, J. (1961). A description and classification of common speech disorders associated with cerebral palsy. *Cerebral Palsy Bulletin, 3,* 57–69.

Irwin, O. C. (1972). *Communication variables of cerebral palsied and mentally retarded children.* Springfield, IL: C. C. Thomas.

Kent, R. D., & Netsell, R. (1975). A case study of an ataxic dysarthric: Cineradiologic and spectrographic observations. *Journal of Speech and Hearing Disorders, 40,* 115–134.

Kent, R. D., & Netsell, R. (1978). Articulatory abnormalities in athetoid cerebral palsy. *Journal of Speech and Hearing Disorders, 43,* 353–373.

Kent, R. D., Netsell, R., & Abbs, J. H. (1979). Acoustic characteristics of dysarthria associated with cerebellar disease. *Journal of Speech and Hearing Research, 22,* 627–648.

Kudrjavcev, T., Schoenberg, B. S., Kurland, L. T., & Groover, R. V. (1983). Cerebral palsy—trends in incidence and changes in concurrent mortality: Rochester, MN, 1950–1976. *Neurology, 33,* 1433–1438.

Leith, W., & Steer, M. (1958). Comparison of judged speech characteristics of athetoids and spastics. *Cerebral Palsy Review, 19,* 15–20.

Lencione, R. (1953). *A study of the speech sound ability and intelligibility status of a group of educable cerebral palsied children.* Unpublished doctoral dissertation, Northwestern University, Evanston, IL.

Lenn, N. J., & Freinkel, A. (1989). Facial sparing in patients with prenatal onset hemiparesis. *Pediatric Neurology, 5,* 291–295.

Little, W. J. (1861). On the influence of abnormal parturition, difficult labour, premature birth, and asphyxia neonatorum on the mental and physical condition of the child, especially in relation to deformities. *Lancet, 2,* 378–380.

Lord, J. (1984). Cerebral palsy: A clinical approach. *Archives of Physical Medicine and Rehabilitation, 65,* 542–548.

Love, R. J., Hagerman, E. L., & Tiami, E. G. (1980). Speech performance, dysphagia and oral reflexes in cerebral palsy. *Journal of Speech and Hearing Disorders, 45,* 59–75.

McDonald, E. T. (1987). Speech production problems. In E. T. McDonald (Ed.), *Treating cerebral palsy* (pp. 1–19). Austin, TX: Pro-ed.

McDonald, E. T., & Chance, B., Jr., (1964). *Cerebral palsy.* Englewood Cliffs, NJ: Prentice-Hall.

Mysak, E. D. (1963). Dysarthria and oropharyngeal reflexology: A review. *Journal of Speech and Hearing Disorders, 28,* 252–260.

Neilson, P. D., Andrews, G., Guitar, B. E., & Quinn, P. T. (1979). Tonic stretch reflexes in lip, tongue and jaw muscles. *Brain Research, 178,* 311–327.

Neilson, P. D., & O'Dwyer, N. J. (1981). Pathophysiology of dysarthria in cerebral palsy. *Journal of Neurology, Neurosurgery and Psychiatry, 44,* 1013–1019.

Neilson, P. D., & O'Dwyer, N. J. (1984). Reproducibility and variability in athetoid dysarthria of cerebral palsy. *Journal of Speech and Hearing Research, 27,* 502–517.

Netsell, R. (1969). Evaluation of velopharyngeal function in dysarthria. *Journal of Speech and Hearing Disorders, 36,* 113–122.

Netsell, R. (1975). *Kinesiology studies of the dysarthrias.* Paper presented at the Workshop on Speech Perception and Production, Stockholm University, Sweden.

Paine, R. S., & Oppe, T. E. (1966). *Neurological examination of children. Clinics in developmental medicine* (Nos. 20/21). London: Spastics Society/Heinemann.

Pharoah, P. O. D., Cooke, T., Rosenbloom, I., & Cooke, R. W. I. (1987). Trends in birth prevalence of cerebral palsy. *Archives of Disease in Childhood, 62,* 379–384.

Platt, L., Andrews, G., & Howie, F. M. (1980). Dysarthria of adult cerebral palsy. II. Phonemic analysis of articulation errors. *Journal of Speech and Hearing Research, 23,* 41–55.

Platt, J. F., Andrews, G., Young, M., & Quinn, P. T. (1980). Dysarthria of adult cerebral palsy. I. Intelligibility and articulatory impairment. *Journal of Speech and Hearing Research, 23,* 28–38.

Riva, D., & Cazzaniga, L. (1986). Late effects of unilateral brain lesions sustained before and after age one. *Neuropsychologia, 24,* 423–428.

Rutherford, B. (1944). A comparative study of loudness, pitch, rate, rhythm and quality of speech of children handicapped by cerebral palsy. *Journal of Speech and Hearing Disorders, 9,* 262–271.

Stark, R. E. (1985). Dysarthria in children. In J. B. Darby (Ed.), *Speech and language evaluation in neurology: Childhood disorders* (pp. 185–217). New York: Grune & Stratton.

Twitchell, T. E. (1961). The nature of the motor deficit in double athetosis. *Archives of Physical Medicine and Rehabilitation, 42,* 63–67.

Westlake, H., & Rutherford, D. R. (1961). *Speech therapy for the cerebral palsied.* Chicago: National Easter Seal Society for Crippled Children and Adults.

Woods, B. T. (1987). Impaired speech shadowing after early lesions of either hemisphere. *Neuropsychologia, 25,* 519–525.

Woods, B. T., & Teuber, H. L. (1973). Early onset of complementary specialization of cerebral hemispheres. *Transactions of the American Neurological Association, 98,* 113–117.

Workinger, M. S., & Kent, R. D. (1991). Perceptual analysis of the dysarthrias in children with athetoid and spastic cerebral palsy. In C. A. Moore, M. M. Yorkston, & D. R. Beukelman (Eds.), *Dysarthria and apraxia of speech* (pp. 109–206). Baltimore: P. H. Brookes.

Yorkston, K. M., & Beukelman, D. R. (1981). *Assessment of intelligibility of dysarthric speech.* Tigard, OR: C. C. Publications.

Yorkston, K. M., Beukelman, D. R., & Bell, K. R. (1988). *Clinical management of dysarthric speakers.* Boston: Little, Brown.

Yorkston, K. M., Beukelman, D. R., Strand, E. A., & Bell, K. R. (1999). *Management of dysarthric speakers in children and adults* (2nd ed.). Austin, TX: Pro-ed.

The Childhood Dysarthrias of the Lower Motor Neuron

If the impairment is caused by a disease of the lower motor neurons, the impairment is said to be peripheral, and if the upper motor neurone, central. The difference between these two types of dysarthria—central and peripheral—have such significant implications in therapy that a few generalizations on the earmarks of each type are in order.
—*ROBERT WEST, MERLE ANSBERRY, AND ANN CARR, 1957*

Introduction
   Motor-Unit Disorders • Incidence • Speech Signs of Lower Motor-Unit Disorders • Clustering of Speech Signs in Flaccid Dysarthria • Neuromuscular Symptoms and Speech Signs • Confirmatory Signs of Lower Motor-Unit Disorder

Lower Motor-Unit Dysarthrias
   Dysarthrias in Disorders of Anterior Horn Cell and Cranial Nerve Motor Neurons • Dysarthrias in Disorders of Peripheral and Cranial Nerve Axons • Dysarthria in Disorders of the Neuromuscular Junction • Dysarthria in Disorders of Muscles

INTRODUCTION

Motor-Unit Disorders

The disorders of the lower motor neurons, or peripheral nervous system, are best understood and classified by employing the concept of the motor unit. This concept provides an explanation of the anatomic sites necessary to classify the neuromuscular diseases of the lower motor neuron. Recall from the discussion in Chapter 2 that the primary sites of the motor unit for diseases with accompanying dysarthrias are

1. the motor nuclei of the upper spinal cord and/or the cranial nerves in the brain stem,
2. the axons of the cranial nerves and upper spinal nerves,
3. the neuromuscular junction of these nerves with muscle, and
4. the muscle fibers themselves.

These anatomic sites are illustrated in Figure 4-1.

Swaiman and Wright (1979) classify the pediatric neuromuscular diseases in terms of both the anatomic site of the pathology and the underlying physiologic disturbance in the lower motor unit. For example, acute anterior bulbar poliomyelitis and Moebius syndrome are disorders of the motor neurons in the spinal cord and/or motor neurons of the cranial nerves in the brain stem. Poliomyelitis is an infectious disease, while Moebius syndrome is congenital.

This combination of the site of lesion with etiology is an attractive classification system, bringing order to an extensive array of neurologic diseases with diverse etiologies. Swaiman and Wright classify the various etiologies of neuromuscular disease as (1) congenital, (2) infectious, (3) toxic, (4) metabolic-degenerative, (5) vascular, and (6) neoplastic. Diseases of the motor unit that commonly present dysarthria and are discussed in this chapter are listed in Table 4-1.

Incidence

Neither the speech-language pathology literature nor the neurology literature is rich in descriptions of the dysarthrias of pediatric neuromuscular disorders. One reason is that the individual motor-unit diseases are much less frequent than are the neuromotor disorders of the upper motor neuron; many of the disorders are considered uncommon in neurology and others are classified as rare. Nonetheless, some of these infrequent disorders have very serious dysarthrias that demand the attention and concern of the speech-language pathologist.

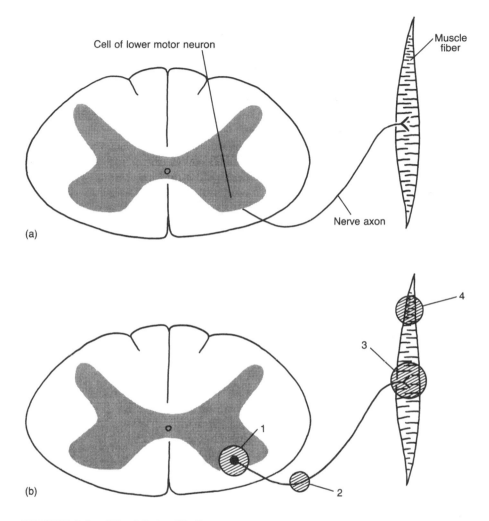

FIGURE 4-1   The Motor Unit
(a) The components of the motor unit, consisting of the cell body of the lower motor neuron, the nerve axon, and the muscle fiber. Lesions at any point in the motor unit will produce signs of a lower motor neuron syndrome. (b) Lesion sites in the motor unit and types of lower motor neuron disorders: (1) cell body (motor neuron disease), (2) lower motor neuron denervation (motor neuropathy), (3) myoneural juncture (neuromyopathy), and (4) muscle fiber (myopathy or dystrophy).

Source: From *Neurology for the Speech-Language Pathologist* (3rd ed.) by R. J. Love and W. G. Webb, 1996, Stoneham, MA: Butterworth Publishers. Copyright 1996 by Butterworth Publishers. Reprinted by permission.

TABLE 4-1   Pediatric Diseases of the Lower Motor Unit That Present Flaccid Dysarthria

Diseases of the anterior horn cell and cranial nerve motor neurons

Juvenile progressive bulbar palsy (Fazio-Londe disease)
Moebius syndrome (congenital facial diplegia)

Diseases of peripheral and cranial nerve axons

Guillain-Barre syndrome
Bell palsy (facial nerve palsy)
Masticator and hypoglossal paralyses
Vocal cord paralysis
Palatal paralysis
Familial dysautonomia (Riley-Day syndrome)

Diseases of the neuromuscular junction

Generalized myasthenia gravis

Diseases of muscle

Duchenne muscular dystrophy
Myotonic dystrophy
Infantile fascioscapulohumeral (FSH) dystrophy
Myopathies

Although accurate prevalence rates are not available for all the pediatric neuromuscular diseases involving a dysarthria, a rough estimate of relative incidence can be established by comparing mean incidence rates of childhood upper motor neuron disorders and lower motor neuron disorders. Pharoah, Cooke, Rosenbloom, and Cooke (1987) have estimated the mean incidence of the most common childhood upper motor neuron disorder, cerebral palsy, as 2.5 cases per 1000 individuals. In contrast, the most common lower motor neuron disorder is Duchenne muscular dystrophy, with an estimated mean incidence of one case per 4425 male live births (Moser, 1984). In this instance, UMN disorders are roughly 10 times as great as LMN disorders in childhood. Further, the pediatric dystrophic population are not as likely to develop a chronic childhood dysarthria as are cerebral-palsied children. Those who do become speech impaired usually do so late in the course of their disease as a result of its progressive nature, while the dysarthria in cerebral palsy is more chronic.

Acute anterior bulbar poliomyelitis, caused by viral involvement of the anterior horn cells in the spinal cord and the homologous cells in the lower brain stem, was once a common cause of childhood lower motor neuron dysarthria. With the advent of the Salk vaccine in 1954 and the attenuated live vaccine in 1960, this dysarthria is very rarely seen in the United States today (Fenichel, 1997). Occasional cases appear in reaction to the vaccine, but they do not constitute a dysarthric population of any size.

Diseases of the neuromuscular juncture are also uncommon in childhood. Myasthenia gravis is the most prevalent of these diseases; however, only about 1% of all patients with myasthenia gravis are children (Teng & Osserman, 1956). The incidence of myastbenia gravis is between 0.5% and 3% per 100,000 population (Kurland & Alter, 1961). Further, fatigability and muscle weakness, the hallmarks of generalized myasthenia gravis, can rapidly be reversed diagnostically by an injection of the drug Tensilon. The diagnosis of a myasthenia thus can be made without referral to a speech-language pathologist for confirmation of the expected bulbar signs of the disease. Moreover, treatment by thymectomy and drug therapy after surgery is usually effective and the speech symptoms are usually relieved or forestalled. The physician often sees no need for referral to the speech-language pathologist for management in most cases.

Other childhood dysarthrias of the motor unit, however, are not as amenable to medical management and demand referral to a speech-language pathologist. A survey of this group of dysarthrias of pediatric neuromuscular disease will follow for the speech-language pathologist, but first the typical dysarthria of motor-unit disorders will be discussed.

Speech Signs of Lower Motor-Unit Disorders

Despite the extensive catalogue of pediatric neuromuscular diseases at their various anatomic sites, the speech signs are similar in all motor-unit disorders, and they all can be classified as a lower motor neuron or **flaccid dysarthria.** The Mayo Clinic classification has popularized the term *flaccid dysarthria* for LMN speech disorders (Darley, Aronson, & Brown, 1975). The original Mayo Clinic research (Darley, Aronson, & Brown, 1969 a & b) identified nine salient deviant speech signs that were recognized in flaccid dysarthria. Listed from most prominent to least prominent, the speech signs are (1) hypernasality, (2) imprecise consonants, (3) continuous breathiness, (4) monopitch, (5) nasal emission, (6) audible inspiration, (7) harsh voice quality, (8) short phrases, and (9) monoloudness. It is well to remember that not all of the nine speech signs will appear in all children with a given neuromuscular disease. For instance, the child who has an involvement of cranial nerve VII, which innervates the facial muscles, will only have minor and transient difficulty with the articulation of bilabial phonemes, while children with severe progressive Duchenne muscular dystrophy may show several deviant speech signs from the list of nine in the later stages of the disease.

Clustering of Speech Signs in Flaccid Dysarthria

The Mayo Clinic research also documented the notion that several combinations of the speech signs may result from an underlying control disturbance of the muscles of the speech mechanism. The research statistically identified three clusters of speech signs that occur in flaccid dysarthria. For instance, the speech signs of nasal emission, imprecise consonants, and hypernasality correlate with short phrases in flaccid dysarthria. These four deviant speech signs form a statistically significant cluster the researchers called **resonatory incompetence.** This cluster was thought to result from a lack of force in muscle contraction and a muscular inability to control closure of the velopharyngeal port.

Two other clusters were statistically derived from the deviant speech signs of flaccid dysarthria. One was called **phonatory incompetence,** which includes breathiness, audible inspiration, and short phrases. It was assumed to be the result of lack of force of muscle contraction.

The third cluster is **phonatory-prosodic insufficiency.** This cluster includes monotony of pitch (monopitch), monoloudness, and harsh voice. The deviant neurologic muscle sign of hypotonia was thought to be the cause of this cluster.

Neuromuscular Symptoms and Speech Signs

Disorders of the motor unit are traditionally associated with the neuromuscular symptoms of weakness, hypotonia, and fatigability of muscles. **Weakness,** the cardinal symptom of lower motor-unit disease, is defined as reduced strength in a specific muscle or group of muscles (Swaiman & Wright, 1979). When taking a history of the child's problems, weakness of gross musculature is usually indicated for the physician by a report of an inability to achieve motor skills or the loss of motor skills during development. Similarly, the speech-language pathologist may find suggestions of fine muscle weakness in case histories of children with congenital neuromuscular disease when there are reports of early feeding problems and excessive drooling.

Both physicians and speech-language pathologists are concerned with weakness in neuromuscular disorders. A **weak muscle** is defined as one that is incapable of contracting to a desired strength and then relaxing, while **normal muscle** is capable of contracting and maintaining a contraction for a considerable time against resistance. The physician tests for weakness by having patients contract muscles in the trunk and limbs and then hold the contraction against resistance. For example, the physician may ask the patient to flex his arm muscles at the elbow joint, contracting his biceps muscle; then the physician will attempt to extend the arm by pulling at the wrist and asking the patient to keep the arm flexed. If the physician can easily extend the arm from the flexed position, weakness may be assumed.

Similarly the speech-language pathologist may assess weakness in the lips, face, tongue, jaw, and velopharynx. Movements of the lips and tongue may be tested for strength by using a tongue blade to provide resistance against tongue and lip movements. Weakness of the muscles of the velopharynx can be inferred by direct observation of the palatopharyngeal muscles. Unilateral palatal weakness can be inferred by determining if there is an asymmetrical elevation of the palatal arches when the velum is raised. Slow or inadequate elevation of both palatal arches usually indicates bilateral weakness of the velum. Jaw opening may be resisted with the hand and weakness of the jaw depressors can be established if the mouth cannot be opened against moderate resistance.

A second critical symptom of neuromuscular disease is fatigue. **Fatigue** is an inability to perform a sustained repetitive motor act. Some children with motor-unit disorders do not demonstrate weak muscles but seem to experience a lack of stamina in sustaining motor acts. For the speech-language pathologist, abnormal fatigue of muscles in the speech mechanism can be tested by asking the child to produce sustained diadochokinetic syllable rates (alternate motion rates for syllables) involving different articulators. Poorly sustained rates suggest abnormal muscle fatigue.

Hypotonia, or reduction of normal muscle tone, is a third major symptom of diseases of the motor unit. Hypotonia generally accompanies significant degrees of weakness, but it may be present in the absence of weakness. The classic method for demonstrating hypotonia is to show reduced resistance to passive movements. A physician usually attempts to determine hypotonia by moving a limb through a full range of motion. Lowered resistance to passive movement accompanied by flabby or flaccid muscles suggests hypotonia.

Hypotonia also can be observed in the oral muscles. The lips may look flaccid and offer no resistance when manipulated with a tongue blade. The lips also may be held habitually in an open mouth posture.

The hypotonic tongue offers little resistance to the tongue blade and lies flaccidly in the mouth. Lingual consonantal contacts are not normally forceful during articulation. There is often a breathy quality in the explosive phase of the production of stop consonants produced with the tongue.

If the vocal folds are flaccid, air escapage at the glottal level is excessive, and there is a continuous breathy quality throughout connected speech. When the child is asked to cough vigorously, the response may be weak.

Weak thoracic muscles may produce a reduction in vocal intensity that results in a soft voice. Thoracic weakness and the resultant soft voice may increase the perception of breathiness.

Confirmatory Signs of Lower Motor-Unit Disorder

In addition to weakness, fatigue, and hypotonia in muscles, the physician will attempt to confirm the diagnosis of lower motor neuron disorder by eliciting other evidence of LMN disturbance. Confirmatory signs of lower motor disorder include diminished or absent tendon reflexes, lack of a Babinski sign, flaccid limb paralysis, lack of clonus, and presence of atrophy. On occasion fasciculations or abnormal muscle twitchings will be seen in muscles, particularly the tongue. In infants, however, fasciculations are usually not detectable in muscles other than the tongue because of overlying subcutaneous fat.

Not all childhood neuromuscular diseases are accompanied by a speech disorder, but some of the well-known motor-unit diseases show specific regional muscle abnormalities that might predispose a child to dysarthria. Some lower motor-unit neuromuscular diseases are specifically characterized by facial and sometimes tongue involvement. Facial weakness is often seen in infantile facioscapulohumeral (FHS) dystrophy, Moebius syndrome, myotonic dystrophy, myopathy, and some forms of muscular dystrophy. In addition to facial weakness, atrophy and fasciculations most often occur in infantile facioscapulohumeral dystrophy (Fenichel, 1997).

LOWER MOTOR-UNIT DYSARTHRIAS

Dysarthrias in Disorders of Anterior Horn Cell and Cranial Nerve Motor Neurons

Dysarthria may be seen in neuromuscular diseases involving the anterior horn cells and the motor neurons of the cranial nerves in the lower brain stem. Following are descriptions of diseases often involving speech problems.

Juvenile Progressive Bulbar Palsy (Fazio-Londe Disease).   Fazio-Londe disease is usually considered a rare motor neuron disease limited to the bulbar muscles. Most cases are sporadic, but heredofamilial cases are reported; no specific mode of genetic transmission has been generally accepted (Fenichel, 1997).

The age of onset is usually between 10 and 20 years, but onset may occur earlier (Gomez, Clermont, & Bernstein, 1962). Initial symptoms usually include facial paralysis, dysphagia, and flaccid dysarthria, although two females, ages 17 and 20, with the presenting symptom of deafness in addition to facial paralysis and dysarthria have been reported (Brucher, Dom, Lombaert, & Carton, 1981). These two cases have been labeled progressive pontobulbar palsy with sensorineural deafness with autosomal recessive inheritance. They may represent a distinct genetic syndrome, one that should be separated from juvenile progressive palsy.

All of the lower cranial nerve nuclei may be affected in juvenile progressive bulbar palsy, but the ocular motor nerve is spared in most cases. Signs of the disease are progressive hypernasality—usually an initial feature—later accompanied by dysphagia, plus facial and tongue weakness. Bulbar atrophy is sometimes severe but often is not present. Fasciculations are not always observed. The course of the disease is fluctuating, but the dysarthria is typically flaccid (Albers, Zimnowodzki, Lowery, & Miller, 1983). Children who show these symptoms along with a rapidly developing progressive motor neuron disease affecting the face and limbs have often been considered to have a childhood form of amyotrophic lateral sclerosis (ALS) rather than a juvenile progressive bulbar palsy (Fenichel, 1997). Thus, a differential diagnosis must be made among myasthenia gravis, ALS, and possibly progressive pontobulbar palsy with deafness. No reports by speech-language pathologists are available in the speech-language pathology literature on this disease.

Moebius Syndrome (Congenital Facial Diplegia). Moebius syndrome, like Fazio-Londe disease, is rare, but it has attracted the attention of speech-language pathologists because of the strong likelihood of a speech disorder. The syndrome is generally characterized by a congenital bilateral facial paralysis of cranial nerve VII (facial diplegia) with abducent nerve (VI) paralyses. Involvement of other cranial nerves, ocular ptosis (dropped eyelid), and muscle deformities have been reported. The etiology is unclear. There are reports of familial incidence in a small number of cases. Pathological studies usually report a **hypoplasia** (lack of tissue development) of brainstem nuclei or cranial nerves, but interuterine disturbances of the brain stem such as vascular malformations or infarctions must also be considered as possible causes (Sudarshan & Goldie, 1985). With a complete paralysis of face and eye muscles, Moebius syndrome is usually evident immediately after birth when the infant has difficulty nursing and closing its eyes. If there is partial paralysis, the problem may not be noted until it is observed that the facial muscle actions are abnormal during laughing and crying. Meyerson and Fourshee (1978) reported that in 22 Moebius syndrome cases, the majority showed an expected flaccid paralysis. There was limited strength and speed in the muscles of articulation. The range of severity of articulation defect was wide. Mild distortions of bilabial phonemes and phonemes requiring tongue-tip elevation were sometimes present. Other subjects showed unintelligible speech. Feeding problems were reported in approximately a third of the patients. Hearing loss, delays in language, and mental retardation were also found. Kahane (1979), reporting on the findings in a single case, found lack of bilabials because of lip paralysis, lingual phoneme substitutions, lack of tongue movement in production of lingualvelar phonemes, and vowel distortion because of imprecise tongue placement.

Dysarthrias in Disorders of Peripheral and Cranial Nerve Axons

A peripheral nerve is composed of axons that originate from motor cell bodies in the central nervous system or from sensory or autonomic ganglia outside the central nervous system. Motor and autonomic fibers make up the anterior or ventral nerve root to the spinal cord. Sensory fibers make up the posterior or dorsal root. The anterior and posterior roots join to form the peripheral nerve containing axons of differing functions. Likewise, the cranial nerves for speech originate from cell bodies in the brain stem of the central nervous system and are composed of several axons that are made up of sensory, motor, and autonomic fibers. Unlike the spinal nerves, not all cranial nerves are mixed in sensory and motor functions. Some are primarily sensory, some are primarily motor, and some are mixed sensory and motor in function.

The cell bodies in the spinal cord and the brain stem are the anatomic sites for maintaining the viability of the axons of the spinal nerves and cranial nerves. Several diseases can affect these two sets of nerves of the peripheral nervous system. The nerve axon, the myelin sheath, or the interstitial connective tissue may be affected by disease. All three sites may be involved in a given disease. The term **neuropathy** signifies a disorder of nerve function without regard for etiologic or pathologic features. The term **neuritis** is used when the disorder is inflammatory in origin. If more than one nerve is involved, the term **polyneuropathy** is used.

The two cardinal characteristics of peripheral nerve involvement are weakness and sensory impairment. The sensory impairment may be either in superficial sensation (touch, pain, and temperature) or in deep sensation (vibration and position sense) or both. Some neuromuscular diseases of the peripheral nerve in which the speech-language pathologist may be summoned as consultant are the following.

Guillain-Barre Syndrome.   This disease is described as an idiopathic neuropathy. It was first reported in the nineteenth century, but its etiology is not yet known. It is presumed to be infectious in origin, and it has been generally associated with a viral infection and autoimmunologic responses. Both children and adults are affected, but onset is usually in adulthood (Juncos & Beal, 1987). The peak incidence for the disease in children occurs between 4 and 10 years. The disease manifests itself in a specific pattern: paralysis often follows a nonspecific infection. There is diffuse lower motor-unit paralysis, either rapid or gradual in onset, with generally symmetrical involvement. Sensory loss may be present, but it is generally less severe than is motor weakness.

Cranial nerve involvement is said to occur in half of the childhood cases (Fenichel, 1997). Bilateral paralysis of the facial nerve (VII) is the most common, but other nerves sometimes are involved. Dysphagia, with particular involvement of cranial nerves IX and X, has been reported in a small number of cases. Respiratory function may be impaired because of weak breathing muscles. The general prognosis is good, with 65% of the patients recovering completely. The remainder show persistent weakness and atrophy of the feet and leg muscles.

The speech-language pathologist may be called upon to perform a dysphagia evaluation or to evaluate the effects of respiratory weakness on speech. A temporary alternate communication system may be instituted during the period of recovery, if needed.

Bell Palsy (Facial Nerve Palsy).   Bell palsy is the result of involvement of the facial nerve (VII). There may be a partial or complete paralysis of one side of the face. In children there is often a mild upper respiratory infection before the onset of the paralysis, with the etiology being an autoimmune reaction (Katusic, Beard, Wiederholt, Bergstralh, & Kurkland, 1986). Pain is often localized to the ear on the affected side. The paralysis may appear suddenly and progress rapidly. The parents often note that the child's face is pulled to one side, while opposite the affected side is flat and immobile. The child will have difficulty closing the eye, drinking, and eating on the affected side. In a complete paralysis the affected side of the face sags, and there is excessive tearing. A mild dysarthria may result from slurring of the bilabial phonemes. In addition, the child may complain of increased auditory activity or special sensitivity to low-frequency sounds on the affected side. In this case, a referral to an audiologist is in order to assess the involvement of the acoustic reflexes with tympanometry. Drug treatment and surgical management have been used in cases of idiopathic facial paralysis. Some cases resolve themselves spontaneously. Approximately 60% of Bell palsy cases have been reported to improve either with treatment or spontaneously. The remainder of patients usually show facial nerve degeneration with long-lasting effects of paralysis (Katusic et al., 1986).

Masticator and Hypoglossal Paralyses.   The muscles of chewing are innervated by cranial nerve V (trigeminal). Isolated paralysis of V is rarely seen unilaterally in children (Darley et al., 1975). Isolated nerve damage is uncommon in cranial nerve XII. When it does occur, the resulting isolated hypoglossal paralysis is marked by unilateral atrophy and fasciculations of the tongue.

Vocal Cord Paralysis.   Damage to the vagus nerve (X) in children is associated with some degree of vocal cord paralysis, which in turn results in a flaccid dysphonia. Vagal paralysis of either the right or left nerve may cause
fixation of the corresponding vocal fold either near the midline or in an adducted position. The paralysis may be congenital or acquired. Acquired conditions such as trauma, growths, or inflammatory illness may affect the
vagus nerve. The symptoms of the flaccid vocal fold near the midline or in
the paramedian position are harshness and reduced loudness. If the cord is
fixed in an adducted position, the voice will be harsh and breathy as well as
reduced in loudness. In addition, **diplophonia** (double vibration in the vocal mechanism), short phrases, and inhalatory stridor will be heard (Darley
et al., 1975). The paralysis may be bilateral, affecting both vocal cords. A midline fixation of the vocal cords produces not only stridor but also difficulty
in breathing for which a tracheostomy may be recommended.

The actual incidence of childhood vocal cord paralysis is unknown, but
Holinger, Holinger, and Holinger (1976) reviewed 389 cases of partial or
complete bilateral adductor vocal cord paralysis. Almost 38% were children
12 years or under. In over half of the children the paralysis was congenital,
while the remaining cases were acquired. Despite the neurologic context,
most of these cases are seen by a laryngologist rather than a neurologist.

Palatal Paralysis.   Unilateral lesions of cranial nerve X often result in weakness of the palate and pharynx as well as the vocal folds, Severe weakness of
the palatopharyngeal muscles will result in dysfunction of the velopharyngeal port. In mild cases, hypernasality results, and in more severe cases, hypernasality and audible nasal emission are present.

In unilateral flaccid paralysis, the affected side of the soft palate reveals
a palatal arch that is on a lower level than is the unaffected side. On phonation, the unaffected side of the palate moves upward easily, while the affected side shows little or no movement. The gag reflex may be modified in
a unilateral paralysis of the palate. There may be little or no elevation of the
soft palate when the gag is stimulated. In bilateral flaccid paralysis or paresis of the muscles of the soft palate, the two palatal arches will rest at a lower
level than will the arches of a normal soft palate. The symmetry of the arches
can give an initial impression of normalcy, except for a slight flattening of the
curvature of the palatal arches. The extent of elevative movement will be reduced on phonation, and the gag reflex will be diminished or absent (Love
& Webb, 1996).

Familial Dysautonomia (Riley-Day Syndrome).   The fundamental defect
in the Riley-Day syndrome is thought to be an imbalance between the
parasympathetic and sympathetic portions of the autonomic nervous system. The syndrome, seen predominantly but not exclusively in Jewish chil-

dren, is characterized by dysphagia from birth, failure to produce an overflow of tears, absent corneal reflexes, hypoactive or absent tendon reflexes, moderate hypotonia, poor motor coordination, postural hypotension, emotional lability, relative indifference to pain, and absence of papillae on the tongue. The disease is genetic, but the mode of inheritance is not always clear (Axelrod, Porges, & Sein, 1987).

The absent corneal reflexes, the relative indifference to pain, and the absence of the taste buds all point to a peripheral sensory defect. The absent or depressed tendon reflexes and the hypotonia can be explained by an interruption of the sensory arc of the stretch reflex. Insufficiency of acetylcholine (Ach), a neurotransmitter at the synapse, has been suggested as the basic mechanism of the disease. There is often a focal demyelinization of the posterior columns of the spinal cord and myelin degeneration of the dorsal roof fibers. This makes it primarily a disease of the sensory roots of the peripheral nerves.

Few reports are available on the dysarthria of children with familial dysautonomia. In 1956, de Hirsch and Jansky reported on 12 children (3 years, 6 months to 12 years, 10 months) examined over a period of time. Delay in onset of the first word was reported in 7 children, and the delayed onset of phrasal usage was found in 8 children. Lip and tongue movement were abnormal in most children. Diadochokinetic oral movements were slowed in 10 children, and drooling was a problem in 11 children. Only 6 children had difficulty with velar movement. Nine children were hypernasal, and 10 were judged to have poor voice quality. Monotonous pitch, poor loudness control, rate abnormalities, and rhythm disturbances were present. Six children had defective articulation for age. The motor speech disorder was judged to be hypotonic, and the speech and voice disturbances can be judged a flaccid dysarthria. Beyond the developmental dysarthria, language disturbances (both in production and comprehension) were found.

The prognosis in familial dysautonomia is poor. Treatment is symptomatic (Fenichel, 1997). Drugs that improve acetylcholine function produce transient relief of some symptoms. Longevity has increased because of improved symptomatic treatment.

Dysarthria in Disorders of the Neuromuscular Junction

The next important anatomic site in the lower motor unit associated with childhood neuromuscular disease is the neuromuscular junction. This is the point where the nerves of the peripheral nervous system—both the cranial and the spinal nerves—synapse with the muscles. Nerve impulses must travel across the synaptic gap from nerve to muscle. Thus the neuromuscular junction is a critical point for important neuromuscular transmission.

Neuromuscular transmission across the synapse is essentially a matter of chemical transmission. The well-known chemical neurotransmitter, acetylcholine (Ach), is responsible for the transmission of electrical impulses. Acetylcholine release at the synapse acts to change the direction of electrical depolarization at the synapse and allows electrical impulses to be generated along muscle fibers from the peripheral nerve.

Generalized Myasthenia Gravis.   Generalized myasthenia gravis is the major disease of the neuromuscular junction. It occurs as the result of a failure in transmission because of reduced availability of acetylcholine at the junction. Antibodies decrease the number of acetylcholine receptors on the postsynaptic membrane in what is called an **autoimmune reaction**. The result is a disorder in which the child shows muscle weakness after sustained muscle contraction. The muscles of the speech mechanism may become affected as well as other muscles of the body. The vagus nerve (X) is sometimes the first to be affected by the disease. Hypernasality may be the first feature in the disease because of involvement of palatopharyngeal muscles (Wolski, 1967). Weakness in other bulbar musculature will follow. Involvement of the speech mechanism is very common in children with generalized myasthenia gravis, but fatigability and weakness are also prime signs in the skeletal muscles.

As indicated earlier, disease of the neuromuscular junction is uncommon in children; only 1% of all patients with myasthenia gravis are children. Fatigability is the cardinal symptom of the disease. Children weaken rapidly with exercise, and symptoms worsen during the day. Early signs include unilateral or bilateral ptosis (eyelid droop), strabismus (crosseyedness), dysphagia, and respiratory difficulties. Speech-language pathologists may play a limited role in treatment, because medical approaches are most effective. To control myasthenic symptoms, thymectomy is done and drug therapy is instituted.

Dysarthria in Disorders of Muscles

The last anatomic site in the classification of neuromuscular diseases of the motor unit is the muscle itself. Disorders of muscle may be divided into two general classes: the dystrophies and the myopathies. The criteria for classifying a muscle disease as a dystrophy or a myopathy are imprecise.

General myopathies are considered primary diseases of striated muscle in which the biochemical, morphologic, or neurophysiologic changes occur singly or in combination (Swaiman & Wright, 1979).

Dystrophies, on the other hand, are hereditary myopathies characterized by progressive muscle degeneration and weakness. They have been grouped together historically and clinically, but they cannot be precisely delineated or classified because little is known of the specific biochemical, physiological, or morphological defects. The dystrophies are discussed first.

Duchenne Muscular Dystrophy. Several types of muscular dystrophy are recognized, but the most common and most severe type is Duchenne muscular dystrophy, named after the French neurologist who first described it in 1861. It is transmitted by X-linked inheritance and affects boys almost exclusively. Typically, its onset is between the ages of 2 and 5 years, and it progresses rapidly. Few patients survive into their early twenties. The disease is found in 1 in every 4425 male live births, and the prevalence is 50,000 in the United States (Muscular Dystrophy Association, 1985). In 1987 it was reported that a protein, dystrophin, is lacking in individuals with Duchenne muscular dystrophy. This protein helps trigger muscular contraction; the absence of the protein ultimately results in a series of events in the muscle cells leading to their destruction and the subsequent loss of muscle strength.

Duchenne dystrophy is marked by a muscle weakness starting in the muscles of the pelvis and trunk and progressing to involvement of all striated muscles, including those used for speech. The visceral muscles are usually spared. A significant diagnostic sign is enlargement of the calf muscle as well as other muscle groups. Infiltration of fat and connective tissue replaces muscle fiber and gives the illusion of increased muscle bulk. This illusion is called **pseudohypertrophy** and explains why Duchenne dystrophy is also called pseudohypertrophic muscular dystrophy.

In the last stages of the disease, a flaccid dysarthria may appear. The articulation disorder is usually mild, often characterized by errors on only one or two phonemes. Dystrophic subjects may show reduced oral breath pressure and vocal intensity. Sanders and Perlstein (1965) have reported that dystrophic subjects do not sustain phonation as well as do normal individuals, and they show serious involvement of the speech musculature. The strength of the tongue and the rate of tongue movements are poor. Pointing and narrowing of the tongue is limited, and pursing and retracting the lips is difficult for the child. In advanced cases, a broadening and flattening of the tongue is often noted. As the disease progresses, respiratory, laryngeal, and pharyngeal muscles all weaken. Labial phonemes are generally produced more correctly than are tongue-tip phonemes. An alternate communication device may be effective in the later stages of the disease to preserve social interaction.

Myotonic Dystrophy. Myotonic dystrophy is an autosomal dominant progressive muscular disorder with variable penetrance that usually becomes apparent in adolescence or later life. The incidence of the disease has been estimated between 2.4 and 4.9 per 100,000 persons (Rowland & Layzer, 1971).

Myotonia is marked by an abnormal persistence of induced or voluntary muscular contraction. The child is unable to relax a contracted muscle quickly or to release a gripped object rapidly. Generally, myotonia affects the distal part of the limb muscles, but also the extraocular, facial, and pharyngeal muscles. Facial muscle atrophy produces similar-looking facies. Problems seen in the neonatal period include impaired swallowing and suckling. There may be facial paralysis (facial diplegia) and arthogyposis (congenital contractures of the joints of the arms and legs). The facial paralysis may be misdiagnosed as a Moebius syndrome. Early sucking and swallowing difficulties may resolve themselves, but the facial paralysis may remain into the second year, and a loss of muscle bulk may cause hollowing of the temporal muscles of the head.

The "myopathic facies" is very common in myotonic dystrophy. Atrophy of the facial muscles gives the patient a long, lean appearance and an expressionless face (Merritt, 1973). Beyond the elongated face, there may be eyelid ptosis, flaccid facial musculature, and an open bite. Neurologic authorities describe speech difficulties and a tendency toward intellectual retardation. Recently, Salomonson, Kawamoto, and Wilson (1988) reported velopharyngeal incompetence as a presenting symptom of myotonic dystrophy in three teenage boys. All three had hypernasality, and one boy had exhibited hypernasal speech from the time he had begun speaking. Treatment consisted of a speech appliance in one case and a superior pharyngeal flap in another. In the third case, traditional speech therapy seemed to be assisted by drug therapy using Diphenylhydantoin. Salomonson et al. (1988) believe that myotonic dystrophy cases initially are best managed nonsurgically. They also point out that velopharyngeal incompetence and hypernasal speech are common presenting symptoms in diseases of the lower motor unit.

Infantile Facioscapulohumeral (FSH) Muscular Dystrophy.   This uncommon disorder was originally considered a muscular dystrophy with autosomal dominant inheritance, but it is currently recognized that children with a genetic facioscapulohumeral weakness also have evidence of myopathy, neuropathy, and inflammation. Although predominantly a dystrophy, this syndrome also shows elements of denervation (Fenichel, 1997).

The onset of weakness is usually in adolescence but may begin in infancy. Initial motor involvement is usually in the shoulder girdle and later spreads to the face; but the reverse may also occur (Bailey, Marzulo, & Hans, 1986). The progression of the muscle weakness is often slow, but eventually there is a change in facial expression.

In the family reported by Bailey et al. (1986), four of eight family members were afflicted, all with an onset from infancy to 5 years. Each developed a severe weakness that led to death in adolescence. Facial weakness and unilateral or bilateral ptosis were common. Hypernasal speech, bulbar muscle weakness, and respiratory insufficiency were present to varying degrees in afflicted family members. Unilateral sensorineural hearing loss at 4000 Hz and above was reported in only one child, although previous reports of this syndrome have indicated that hearing loss is commonly associated with the disorder.

No account of speech intervention has been reported in this form of muscular dystrophy, to my knowledge. Mabis, Webb, & Love (1976) reported successful use of a palatal lift to reduce hypernasality and velopharyngeal incompetence in a related syndrome of muscular dystrophy—occulopharyngeal muscular dystrophy. Typically, onset of bulbar signs in this dystrophic syndrome is limited to adults (Little & Perl, 1982), as was the case in our report of dysarthria management by palatal lift.

Myopathies. The myopathies are diseases of abnormal changes in the muscle itself or the membranes of the muscle. The predominating symptom is muscle weakness. If the myopathy is congenital, the infant is characterized by hypotonia with a subsequent development of progressive proximal and symmetrical muscular weakness. Several myopathies have their onset later in childhood. Some of the congenital myopathies are associated with a dominant inheritance pattern, while others are associated with a recessive inheritance, and still others have been described with different forms of inheritance.

Myopathies are sometimes characterized by the presence of specific cranial nerve deficits, and if cranial nerves innervating the bulbar muscles are involved, speech functions may be disturbed. Since these myopathies are quite rare, there is not yet any speech pathology literature concerning their diagnoses, evaluation, or management. The speech-language pathologist faced with such a case is advised to consult a standard textbook of pediatric neuromuscular diseases to determine the specific nature of the myopathic disease and then proceed with a speech evaluation, expecting the traditional symptoms of a flaccid dysarthria.

SUMMARY

The childhood dysarthrias of the lower motor neuron are much less common than are those of the upper motor neuron, such as the dysarthrias of cerebral palsy. In fact, many of the LMN dysarthrias are uncommon or even rare. The cerebral palsies are roughly 10 times more frequent.

Lower motor neuron disorders can be anatomically classified by lesion sites at various points in the lower motor unit. Lesions in the anterior horn cells of the spinal cord or motor nuclei of the brain stem include progressive bulbar palsy (Fazio-Londe disease) and Moebius syndrome. Lesions of the peripheral cranial nerve are associated with Guillain-Barre syndrome, Bell palsy, vocal cord paralysis, palatal paralysis, and familial dysautonomia (Riley-Day syndrome). Myasthenia gravis, a rare disorder in children, is associated with a lesion at the neuromuscular junction.

Lesions in the muscles produce a dystrophy or a myopathy. Of the dystrophies associated with a dysarthria, the following are most important in speech pathology: Duchenne muscular dystrophy, myotonic dystrophy, and infantile facioscapulohumeral (FSH) muscular dystrophy. Dysarthrias in the congenital myopathies have not been reported in the speech pathology literature.

Important signs of lower motor-unit disorder in children include weakness, fatigability, hypotonia, atrophy, and fasciculations, except in individual nerve palsies of V, VII, X, and XII, where weakness and paralysis dominate. Hypernasality often is the major presenting speech sign in LMN disorders. Its basis is velopharyngeal dysfunction. Major speech signs of flaccid dysarthria, in addition to hypernasality, include imprecise consonants, continuous breathiness, nasal emission, audible expiration, harsh voice, short phrases, and monopitch.

SUGGESTED READING

Darley, F. L., Aronson, A. E., & Brown, J. R. (1975). Flaccid dysarthria: Disorders of the lower motor neuron. *Motor speech disorders* (pp. 99–128). Philadelphia: W. B. Saunders.

A complete treatment of flaccid dysarthria in the adult. The basic findings can also be applied to the childhood dysarthrias of neuromuscular diseases.

Fenichel, G. M. (1997). *Clinical pediatric neurology* (3rd ed.). Philadelphia: W. B. Saunders.

This book, by an expert in pediatric neuromuscular diseases, gives clear and complete descriptions of LMN diseases and their medical treatment.

Salomonson, J., Kawamoto, H., & Wilson, L. (1988). Velopharyngeal incompetence as the presenting symptom of myotonic distrophy. *Cleft Palate Journal, 25,* 296–300.

This article discusses dysarthria in myotonic dystrophy and suggests that velopharyngeal incompetence may be the presenting symptom of all the disorders of speech of the lower motor unit in children.

Swaiman, K. F., & Wright, F. S. (1979). *Pediatric neuromuscular disease.* St. Louis, MO: C. V. Mosby.

This standard neurologic textbook is difficult reading, but it provides a very comprehensive survey of the lower motor-unit disorders in a clear and organized manner.

REFERENCES

Albers, J. W., Zimnowodzki, S., Lowery, C., & Miller, B. (1983). Juvenile progressive bulbar palsy: Clinical and electrodiagnostic findings. *Archives of Neurology, 40,* 351–353.

Axelrod, F. B., Porges, R. F., & Sein, M. E. (1987). Neonatal recognition of familial dysautonima. *Journal of Pediatrics, 110,* 946–948.

Bailey, R. O., Marzulo, D. C., & Hans, M. B. (1986). Infantile facioscapulohumeral muscular dystrophy: New observations. *Acta Neurologica Scandinavia, 74,* 51–58.

Brucher, J. M., Dom, R., Lombaert, A., & Carton, H. (1981). Progressive pontobulbar palsy with deafness: Clinical and pathological study of two cases. *Archives of Neurology, 38,* 186–190.

Darley, F. L., Aronson, A. E., & Brown, J. R. (1969a). Differential diagnostic patterns of dysarthria. *Journal of Speech and Hearing Research, 12,* 246–269.

Darley, F. L., Aronson, A. E., & Brown, J. R. (1969b). Clusters of deviant speech dimensions in the dysarthrias. *Journal of Speech and Hearing Research, 12,* 462–496.

Darley, F. L., Aronson, A. E., & Brown, J. R. (1975). *Motor speech disorders.* Philadelphia: W. B. Saunders.

de Hirsch, K., & Jansky, J. J. (1956). Language investigation of children suffering from familial dysautonomia. *Journal of Speech and Hearing Disorders, 21,* 450–460.

Fenichel, G. M. (1997). *Clinical pediatric neurology.* (3rd ed.). Philadelphia: W. B. Saunders.

Gomez, M., Clermont, V., & Bernstein, J. (1962). Progressive bulbar paralysis in children (Fazio-Londe disease). *Archives of Neurology, 6,* 317–323.

Holinger, L. D., Holinger, P. C., & Holinger, P. H. (1976). Etiology of bilateral adductor vocal cord paralysis. A review of 289 cases. *Annals of Otology, Rhinology and Laryngology, 85,* 428–436.

Juncos, J. L., & Beal, M. F. (1987). Idiopathic cranial polyneuropathy. A fifteen year experience. *Brain, 110-1,* 197–211.

Kahane, J. (1979). Pathophysiological effects of Moebius syndrome on speech and hearing. *Archives of Otolaryngology, 105,* 29–34.

Katusic, S. K., Beard, C. M., Wiederholt, W. C., Bergstralh, E. J., & Kurkland, L. T. (1986). Incidence, clinical features and progress in Bell's palsy, Rochester, Minnesota, 1968–1982. *Annals of Neurology, 20,* 622–629.

Kurland, L. T., & Alter, M. (1961). Current status of the epidemiology and genetics of myasthenia gravis. In H. R. Viets (Ed.), *Myasthenia gravis.* Springfield, IL: Charles C. Thomas.

Little, B. W., & Perl, D. P. (1982). Oculopharyngeal muscular dystrophy. *Journal of the Neurological Sciences, 53,* 145–158.

Love, R. J., & Webb, W. G. (1996). *Neurology for the speech-language pathologist* (3rd ed.). Stoneham, MA: Butterworth.

Mabis, J. H., Webb, W. G., & Love, R. J. (1976, November). *Use of a palatal lift in oculopharyngeal muscular dystrophy.* Paper presented at the annual convention of the American Speech-Language-Hearing Association, Houston, TX.

Merritt, H. H. (1973). *A textbook of neurology.* Philadelphia: Lea and Febiger.

Meyerson, M., & Fourshee, D. (1978), Speech, language and hearing in Moebius syndrome. *Developmental Medicine and Child Neurology, 20,* 357–365.

Moser, H. (1984). Duchenne muscular dystrophy: Pathogenic aspects and genetic prevention. *Human Genetics, 66,* 17–22.

Muscular Dystrophy Association (1985). *Duchenne muscular dystrophy.* New York: Muscular Dystrophy Association, 1–14.

Pharoah, P. O. D., Cooke, T., Rosenbloom, I., & Cooke, R. W. I. (1987). Trends in birth prevalence of cerebral palsy. *Archives of Disease in Childhood, 62,* 379–384.

Rowland, L. P., & Layzer, R. B. (1971). Muscular dystrophies, atrophies and related disease. In A. G. Baker & L. H. Baker (Eds.), *Clinical neurology.* New York: Harper & Row.

Salomonson, J., Kawamoto, H., & Wilson, L. (1988). Velopharyngeal incompetence as the presenting symptom of myotonic dystrophy. *Cleft Palate Journal, 25,* 296–300.

Sanders, L. J., & Perlstein, M. A. (1965). Speech mechanism in pseudohypertrophic muscular dystrophy. *American Journal of Diseases of Children, 109,* 538–543.

Sudarshan, A., & Goldie, W. D. (1985). The spectrum of congenital facial diplegia (Moebius syndrome). *Pediatric Neurology, 1,* 180–184.

Swaiman, K. F., & Wright, F. S. (1979). *Pediatric neuromuscular diseases.* St. Louis, MO: C. V. Mosby.

Teng, P., & Osserman, K. E. (1956). Studies in myasthenia gravis: Neonatal and juvenile types. A report of 21 and a review of 188 cases. *Journal of Mount Sinai Hospital New York, 23,* 71.

West, R., Ansberry, M., & Carr, A. (1957). *The rehabilitation of speech* (3rd ed.). New York: Harper & Row.

Wolski, W. (1967). Hypernasality as the presenting symptom of myasthenia gravis. *Journal of Speech and Hearing Disorders, 32,* 36–38.

▶ 5

Developmental Verbal Dyspraxia

Developmental articulatory apraxia or dyspraxia . . . has been described as a defect of articulation which occurs when movements for speech, that is of tongue, lips, or palate appear normal for involuntary and spontaneous movement such as smiling or licking the lips, or even for voluntary imitation of movements carried out on request, but are inadequate for the complex and rapid movements used for articulation . . .
—*MURIEL MORLEY, 1957*

Controversial Issues
    Etiology and Pathology • Signs, Symptoms, and Syndromes • Phonologic-Linguistic Variables

Single Case Studies: Evidence for the Disorder
    Type of Evidence in Case Studies

Recent Developments
    The Iowa and Crary Textbooks • The Wisconsin Articles

Developmental verbal dyspraxia (DVD), as suggested in Chapter 1, is widely considered a controversial motor speech diagnosis at many levels. The intent of this chapter is to document the nature of the controversy and to indicate that despite the serious questions raised about the etiology, pathology, and validity of the reported signs and symptoms of the DVD syndrome, it remains an appropriate and useful diagnostic category of childhood motor speech disability.

CONTROVERSIAL ISSUES

Etiology and Pathology

The etiology and pathology of DVD are unknown. Although often it has seemed reasonable to consider DVD in a neurologic context and to seek evidence of brain lesions as etiological explanations similar to those in its adult analogue, there is yet no convincing evidence of localized and lateralized brain lesions similar to those found in the adult, nor is there unequivocal evidence of minor and inconsistent neurologic signs ("soft" signs) in all children studied to date (Darwish, Pearce, Gaines, & Harasym, 1982; Ferry, Hall, & Hicks, 1975; Horwitz, 1984; Love & Fitzgerald, 1984; Rosenbek & Wertz, 1972; Williams, Ingham, & Rosenthal, 1981; Yoss & Darley, 1974a). (See Chapter 2 for a fuller discussion of the neurologic reports on DVD.)

There is some data suggesting heredofamilial tendencies in DVD. Morley (1957), Ferry et al. (1975), Aram and Nation (1982), and Lewis (1990) have all noted family histories of speech and language disorders in the backgrounds of children with suspected DVD. Although reports such as these are highly provocative, they do not provide incontrovertible evidence of genetic etiology in the disorder. However, the lack of clear-cut brain lesion evidence and the suggestion of possible genetic influence as a basis for etiology are not unexpected in childhood speech disorders. It is well-known to neurologists and pediatricians that developmental speech and language disorders do not have specific correlates with brain anatomy as do disorders of adult speech and language (Kirshner, 1986). In fact, Rapin (1988) has summed up the nature of the etiology of childhood disorders of higher cerebral function in these words:

> In most cases the cause is unknown. Prenatal and genetic etiologies seem to predominate over acquired insults to the developing brain as the result of prematurity, perinatal anoxia or trauma and prenatal infections. . . . The fact that boys are affected much more often (4:1) than girls reinforces the probability that exogenous insults of the brain are unlikely to be responsible for the majority of cases. (p. 1119)

In brief, in most cases of children with higher cerebral dysfunctions like DVD, the brain will appear structurally normal, with the exception of minor developmental anomalies, possibly of a genetic origin.

Signs, Symptoms, and Syndromes

Of all the areas of controversy surrounding DVD, the issue of whether the disorder presents itself as a clear and consistent syndrome is probably the most debated. A **syndrome** is a cluster of physical signs and symptoms that indicates a specific disease or disorder, and DVD is usually defined by a syndrome cluster (Aram & Nation, 1982; Hall, Hardy, & LaVelle, 1990; Thompson, 1988). There is, however, confusion in the literature of DVD as to the exact symptom behaviors that should be included in the DVD syndrome cluster. Jaffe (1986) has pointed out that DVD appears to be a syndrome in which all symptoms and signs need not be present to diagnose the disorder, nor must one typical sign or symptom be present to establish the diagnosis.

Further, the commonly reported signs and symptoms of DVD are not exclusive to the disorder but may overlap with symptoms of other speech-disordered populations. Serious skepticism about the validity of a well-defined syndrome designated as DVD was no doubt fueled by the extensive 49-page critical review of the subject by Guyette and Diedrich (1981). Surveying more than 100 publications related to the topic, they pointed out several contradictions, confusions, and scientific design flaws in the clinical and experimental field literature on the subject. Guyette and Diedrich observed that many of the reports of children with DVD were not based on empirical data and that the few data-based reports often presented findings that were at odds with each other and were inconclusive.

In addition, it has been observed that there has been little consistency in criteria for subject selection in DVD studies because of the lack of agreement on a definition of the disorder (Thompson, 1988). Subjects have varied in age, intelligence quotients, and language ability. For instance, children between the ages of 5 and 10 years who demonstrated articulation disorders were studied in two well-known experimental field reports (Yoss & Darley, 1974a; Williams et al., 1981), but in a retrospective study Rosenbek and Wertz (1972) reported on children between 2 and 14 years of age; Ferry et al. (1975) studied subjects up to the age of 30. Intelligence quotient levels have varied along with age in these often-cited reports. Ferry et al. studied subjects with intelligence quotients from 40 to 120. Yoss and Darley as well as Williams et al. selected subjects with IQs of 90 or above. Intelligence levels were not limited by Rosenbek and Wertz in their study, and they made no effort to exclude mentally retarded subjects.

Criteria for the presence or absence of language delay also differed from study to study. Williams et al. (1981) and Yoss and Darley (1974a) selected subjects with a language age of no more than 6 months below chronological age and with no known organic disability. Rosenbek and Wertz (1972) did not exclude subjects with language delay, nor did Ferry et al. (1975).

Symptom Disagreement. The lack of homogeneity in subject selection of children diagnosed as having DVD is indicative of the lack of agreement among authors about which symptoms and signs constitute the disorder. Thompson (1988) has listed signs and symptoms of DVD that have been reported in DVD studies published from 1972 to 1983 (see Table 5-1). Although it is helpful to have reported signs and symptoms presented in an organized manner such as this, Thompson herself offers several cautions about the interpretation of her tabular material. First, many of the signs and symptoms listed were derived from clinical observation and were not studied empirically; authors often present observations with no data to support them (Chappell, 1973; Edwards, 1973; Morley, 1972). Second, the tabular material reflects significant disagreement in the literature about the presence or absence of critical signs and symptoms. In no way does it present a clear-cut diagnostic profile of DVD. Thompson particularly notes disagreement on items such as error consistency, vowel errors, distortions, additions, cluster reduction, articulatory groping, presence or absence of oral apraxia, and language deficits. Despite the serious problems of symptom validity and agreement, Table 5-1 on pages 90–91 suggests that DVD may indeed be a clinical entity different from other speech disorders such as mild developmental dysarthria or developmental phonologic disability of idiopathic etiology.

Admittedly, DVD is currently ill-defined and poorly documented in an empirical sense, but as Love and Fitzgerald (1984) have argued, its recognition and description by Morley (1957) is highly significant, since it established an often unrecognized clinical entity that provides substantial assistance in the differential diagnosis of the most prevalent speech disorder encountered by the speech-language pathologist—a developmental phonologic disorder, or so-called "functional articulation disorder." The appropriate identification of children with phonologic disorders whose etiology is likely neurogenic rather than learned or idiopathic provides added explanatory power to the understanding, assessing, and managing of a select group of children with severe and often unyielding articulation defects that make them special problem cases for the speech-language pathologist. Further, it often explains preschool childhood speech and language delay of so-called developmental aphasia (Daly, Cantrill, Cantrill, & Aman, 1972; Eisenson, 1984; Morley, 1957).

One significant value in correctly diagnosing a child with a DVD syndrome is that the diagnosis often radically changes the direction of therapeutic management and opens the door to a variety of techniques not usually employed with the typical child with developmental phonologic disability or suspected developmental aphasia. These techniques have included oromotor and orosensory training for articulation (Haynes, 1985), special cueing techniques (Bashir, Grahamjones, & Bostwick, 1984; Klick, 1985), visual approaches to speech and language (Shelton & Graves, 1985), augmentative communication via manual sign language in preschoolers (Harlan, 1984), melodic intonation therapy (MIT) (Helfrich-Miller, 1984), and the use of a palatal lift to improve velopharyngeal dysfunction (Hall et al., 1990).

Syndrome Definition.   If the diagnosis of DVD is appropriate and useful in cases of preschool language disorders and in atypical school-age articulation disorders, how can the definition of the syndrome be clarified and strengthened to avoid discarding the whole concept, as Guyette and Diedrich (1981) have recommended? To retain DVD as a viable syndrome, one must first define the disorder in terms of an obvious, widely reported and constant physical sign, without which the diagnosis cannot be made, along with a set of less-fixed symptoms (Love & Fitzgerald, 1984). Grunwell and Yavas (1988) assert that a motor programming disorder of speech has become the widely accepted putative definition of DVD. In other words, a motor speech programming disability is almost unanimously considered the *sine qua non* of DVD (Eisenson, 1984; Hall et al., 1990; Morley, 1957; Rosenbek & Wertz, 1972; Weiner, 1969; Williams et al., 1981; Yoss & Darley, 1974a). The defining motor problem, an inability to consistently position the articulators for speech, may lead to a variety of symptoms—some motor, such as oral diadochokinesis disability; some phonological, such as inconsistent articulatory errors, vowel distortions, consonant omission, and distortion and addition errors; and some linguistic, such as word retrieval and syntactic disability.

We further maintain that the motor programming disorders may disrupt verbal motor performance alone or verbal motor performance may be disrupted because of an underlying developmental oral apraxia (DOA); this is consistent with Yoss and Darley's (1974a) definition of developmental apraxia of speech. In other words, DVD may be present in speech alone or may coexist with nonspeech oral movement problems,

The categories of an isolated verbal dyspraxia and a verbal dyspraxia caused by oral apraxia have been empirically documented and accepted in adult motor speech disorders but have not been completely accepted in childhood disorders (Aram & Nation, 1982; DeRenzi, Pieczuro, & Vignolo, 1966; Morley, 1957; Wertz, LaPointe, & Rosenbek, 1984).

Beyond establishing the necessary and sufficient physical sign of motor programming disability to define the DVD syndrome, it is important to answer the several criticisms of symptom variability as a major threat to the validity of the DVD syndrome (Guyette & Dedrich, 1981; Jaffe, 1984; Thompson, 1988). It is very unlikely when considering the issue of symptom variability that any given child suspected of DVD will fit exactly the symptom picture proposed in any of the specific varied descriptions of the DVD syndrome in the textbook literature. This lack of common symptoms in DVD children is the heart of the controversy concerning the validity of the DVD syndrome. The diagnosis of DVD is not necessarily negated in suspected

TABLE 5-1 Speech and Nonspeech Symptoms Reported in the Literature as Characteristic (or not Characteristic) of Developmental Apraxia of Speech

Presenting symptoms	Characteristic	Not characteristic
Speech Symptoms		
Inconsistent errors	Rosenbek & Wertz (1972); Edwards (1973); Morley (1972)	Yoss & Darley (1974a)
Inability to imitate speech sounds	Chappell (1973); Edwards (1973); Macaluso-Haynes (1978); Rosenbek, Hansen, Baughman, & Lemme (1974)	
Vowel distortion	Rosenbek & Wertz (1972)	Morley (1972); Yoss & Darley (1974a)
Omission errors	Yoss & Darley (1974a); Williams, Ingham, & Rosenthal (1981); Rosenbak & Wertz (1972); Smartt, LaLance, Gray, & Hibbett (1976)	
Distortion errors	Yoss & Darley (1974a); Rosenbek & Wertz (1972)	Williams, Ingham, & Rosenthal (1981); Smartt, LaLance, Gray, & Hibbett (1976)
Addition errors	Yoss & Darley (1974a); Williams, Ingham, & Rosenthal (1981); Rosenbek & Wertz (1972)	Smartt, LaLance, Gray, & Hibbett (1976)
One feature errors	Williams, Ingham, & Rosenthal (1981); Yoss & Darley (1974a)	
Two or three feature errors	Yoss & Darley (1974a); Williams, Ingham, & Rosenthal (1981)	
Prolongations	Yoss & Darley (1974a); Rosenbek & Wertz (1972)	
Repetition errors	Yoss & Darley (1974a); Rosenbek & Wertz (1972)	
Consonant cluster errors	Rosenbek & Wertz (1972)	
Fricative errors	Rosenbek & Wertz (1972)	
Affricate errors	Rosenbek & Wertz (1972)	Yoss & Darley (1974a)

Characteristic	References
Methathetic errors	Edwards (1973); Morley (1972); Rosenbek & Wertz (1972)
Sequencing errors	Chappell (1973); Edwards (1973); Morley (1972); Rosenbek & Wertz (1972)
Articulatory groping	Rosenbek & Wertz (1972); Yoss & Darley (1974a)
Voicing errors	Yoss & Darley (1974a)
Increased errors with increased length and complexity	Rosenbek & Wertz (1972); Edwards (1973)
Prosodic disturbance	Rosenbek & Wertz (1972); Edwards (1973); Yoss & Darley (1974a)
Non-speech Symptoms	
Oral apraxia	Chappell (1973); Rosenbek & Wertz (1972); Yoss & Darley (1974a); Aram (1979); Ferry, Hall, & Hicks (1975); Court & Harris (1965)
Diadochokinetic difficulty	Aram (1979); Yoss & Darley (1974)
Language deficits	Greene (1967); Rosenbek & Wertz (1972); Edwards (1973); Aram (1979); Ekelman & Aram (1983); Williams, Ingham, & Rosenthal (1981); Yoss & Darley (1974a); Chappell (1973)

Adapted with permission. From Thompson, C. K. Articulation disorders in the child with neurogenic pathology. In N. J. Lass, L. V. McReynolds, J. L. Northern, & D. E. Yoder, (Eds.). *Handbook of speech-language pathology and audiology* (pp. 548–591). Toronto: BC Decker, 1988.

cases because the signs and symptoms of the case do not match exactly the reported fixed and consistent textbook descriptions of a syndrome. As neurologist D. Frank Benson (1979) points out, it is quite uncommon to see complete syndromes in neurologic medicine. Syndrome variability often leads to confusion among clinicians about the concept of a syndrome, he notes. Benson observes that many individuals consider a neurologic syndrome to be a completely fixed and invariant group of findings; in other words, each symptom must invariably be present if a specific disorder is to be diagnosed. However, in actuality syndromes are as rare and as uncommon in neurologic medicine as they are in any other branch of medicine. The individual features of a syndrome are not to be considered firm and fixed, and a given syndrome should not be thought of as the inevitable result of either a specific process or of anatomic localization. Only in the broadest sense, Benson states, do the features of a neurologic disorder bunch together into a few comparative consistent clusters called syndromes.

With Benson's admonitions in mind, it appears quite possible to retain the concept of a DVD syndrome if the necessary and sufficient conditions of a voluntary motor programming disorder either at the speech or nonspeech level are met. This motor programming disability may or may not result in a rigidly consistent set of motor, phonologic, linguistic, or neurologic signs or symptoms, and inconsistency among symptoms should be expected as typical rather than atypical.

Phonologic-Linguistic Variables

As the previous discussion of the DVD syndrome suggests, it is quite common for specific DVD symptoms to vary from child to child. Although there may be great individual differences in symptoms or behavioral features, it also may be the case that symptom patterns retain some consistency when large samples of children are surveyed. Faced with uncertainties in the areas of etiology and syndrome definition, speech-language pathologists have recently turned to the study of phonologic-linguistic variables in group research to answer some of the basic questions about the nature of DVD symptoms.

Equated Groups.   One line of research has employed equated group research designs to determine if phonologic features separate children suspected of DVD from children with a developmental phonologic disability. Equated group designs are the preferred research paradigm to determine if two groups vary on a given dimension (Cook & Campbell, 1979). The well-known Yoss and Darley study (1974a), which was highly instrumental in establishing DVD as a possible clinical entity in present-day speech-language pathology, was the first to employ an equated design in which phonologic features were systematically studied. A group of 30 severely and moderately severely misarticulating children between the ages of 5 and 10 years with normal hearing, intelligence, and similar language ability were separated in a well-constructed test of isolated volitional nonspeech oral movements (oral apraxia test) and then tested for phonologic differences. The authors reported that several types of error sounds differentiated the two groups. The oral apraxic group, designated as the developmental apraxia of speech sample, used more phoneme distortions, prolongations, repetitions, and additions in repeated sound tasks than did the matched misarticulating group. Two- and three-feature errors were most likely to occur in children with suspected DAS. In spontaneous speech, a different set of errors emerged as predictive of DAS. These errors included phoneme distortions, one-place feature errors, additions, and omissions. Despite variations in errors according to speech task, clear differences were reported between the two groups. The articulation results, plus soft signs in the DAS group, appeared to establish a clinical entity. The study, at the time of its publication, seemed to offer conclusive evidence that children suspected of DAS could be separated from children with severe developmental phonologic disability.

These important empirical findings, however, were challenged by Williams et al. (1981) in a well-designed replication in which Australian children were studied. Employing a sample of children defined by similar subject variables from the earlier study, except that subjects suspected of DAS were not those seen at a large medical center (Mayo Clinic), Williams et al. (1981) found that children suspected of DAS differed from the equated group on few of the variables being tested. Only 2 of the 11 speech variables differentiated the two groups. Omission errors on repeated speech tasks and omissions in spontaneous speech clearly separated the two groups of misarticulating Australian children. However, if the omission errors were removed from the phonologic samples, differences between the two groups were not obvious at all. It clearly appeared that school-age children with suspected DAS could not be consistently differentiated from equated children with developmental phonologic disability.

A third study employing equated groups confirmed the findings of Williams et al. (1981) concerning the lack of differences in phonologic abilities of these two types of misarticulating children. Parsons (1984) studied the phonologic processes of children suspected of DVD. He used 7 clinical subjects and a control group equated on major subject variables. The age range of the subjects was slightly younger than in the earlier studies, from 4 years, 6 months to 6 years, 8 months. Twenty-four phonologic processes were studied, and statistical analysis of the use of the phonologic processes revealed no significant differences between the two groups. Only two phonologic processes even approached statistical significance. The processes more common in the suspected DVD children were (1) backing of front phonemes and

(2) insertion of sounds or epenthesis. Parsons interpreted his data to mean that the children with suspected DVD are neither a special etiologic group nor a subcategory of developmental phonologic ability. In summary, the results of these three equated group studies are not unanimous. However, the lack of differences in phonologic performance in the more recent studies strongly suggests that children suspected of DVD do not present different phonologic features from the typical misarticulating child with multiple misarticulations.

Unique Phonologic Characteristics.   Researchers who have studied group phonologic characteristics without the benefit of an equated control group or a systematic testing for oral apraxic elements have claimed that children with DVD present unique phonologic characteristics. Crary (1984) summarized a series of studies that he and his colleagues performed on children believed to be verbal apraxics. Crary defined DVD on the basis of oral motor disability, and he used a highly heterogeneous series of samples of oral motor disability in this regard. None of the total population displayed oral motor weakness, but some children displayed "motor incoordination" in their speech mechanisms. A broad sample of children were included who demonstrated "a strong oral apraxia accompanied by postural groping to a selective deficit in lingual elevation" (Crary, 1984, p. 72).

Thirteen phonologic processes were analyzed in a series of studies on children with DVD, as defined by Crary. Syntagmatic processes showed the most errors. These included deletion of initial and final consonants as well as glottal replacement. Factor analysis of the phonologic processes data suggested that the primary factor was omission of phonemes in all syllable positions. Syllable structure control thus appeared to be a major component in the children considered to be DVD cases. Further errors tended to be of sound classes representing more complex articulations.

Interesting as these results are, they must be considered suspect because of the negative results of phonologic differences and phonologic processes reported in the better-designed studies of Williams et al. (1981) and Parsons (1984), who used equated control groups. Crary's results would have been much stronger if appropriate control groups of misarticulating children had been employed and a systematic oral apraxia test had been given.

If indeed certain phonologic processing is typical of children with DVD, further research is needed in this area. There is evidence that there is consistency in use and frequency of phonologic processes under varying linguistic and performance load tasks in the DVD child (Bowman, Parsons, & Morris, 1984). This consistency of phonologic processes needs to be investigated with non-DVD children and then comparisons made with DVD children.

Linguistic Impairment.   Investigators more recently have explored the aspect of language disability in DVD, assuming that the DVD disorder must be more than an oral motor disability and resulting phonologic errors. Panagos and Bobkoff (1984) argue on theoretical grounds that verbal dyspraxia can never be conceived as a limited motor or phonologic problem, because phonology is a quasi-autonomous component of language. Defects that appear to be primarily phonologic always have ramifications for the total linguistic system. Panagos and Bobkoff believe that verbal dyspraxia is a disorder of language encoding that involves cognitive mechanisms more than it does motor mechanisms.

Several authors (Edwards, 1973; Grunwell & Yavas, 1988; Love & Fitzgerald, 1984; Prichard, Tekieli, & Kozup, 1977; Rosenbek & Wertz, 1972; Weiner, 1969) have reported language impairment or delay in DVD children, but the work of Ekelman and Aram (1984) has received considerable attention in this regard. They presented syntactic data on eight children with DVD along with data on syntactic change over time on three of the eight children. The children were diagnosed with DVD on the basis of slowed syllable rates and syllable sequencing, but no oral apraxia test was given. Results of the study showed that all eight children had disordered sentence structure in terms of an expected mean length of utterance for age. Six of the eight children were below expectation for age on Lee's *Developmental Sentence Analysis* procedure (1974). Errors in some grammatical markers were not attributed to motor speech or phonologic limitations completely; a primary language problem was considered to be present. Analysis of syntax change in three subjects indicated improvement over time.

Although the data suggested a significant language disability component in DVD, the study has been criticized on the grounds that oral dyspraxia was not clearly established or denied by oral apraxic testing. Moreover, similar findings of linguistic impairment have been found in nondyspraxic children with multiple misarticulations (Deputy, 1984).

SINGLE CASE STUDIES: EVIDENCE FOR THE DISORDER

Speech-language pathologists who have found group studies of DVD unconvincing because of inconsistent definitions of oral and/or verbal dyspraxia and lack of equivalent non-dyspraxic controls in critical research have turned to the case study approach to provide more compelling evidence for the validity of DVD and to establish the nature of disorder (Grunwell & Yavas, 1988; Love & Fitzgerald, 1984) or to test the efficacy of therapeutic techniques (Daly et al., 1972; Hall et al., 1990; Harlan, 1984; Helfrich-Miller, 1984; Klick, 1985; Rosenbek, Hansen, Baughman, & Lemme, 1974; Shelton &

Graves, 1985; Yoss and Darley, 1974b). The case study approach has been widely used in the health sciences to provide descriptions of unusual cases and to offer new information about poorly understood disorders. On occasion, case studies have clarified controversial issues and have become a starting point for research in new directions (Oyster, Hanten, & Llorens, 1987).

Type of Evidence in Case Studies

Recent single case studies of children with suspected DVD provide compelling evidence for the diagnosis and use of the concept of DVD. First, some reported cases have been observed longitudinally for several years, allowing the speech-language pathologist to determine over time whether the case under study fits the expected clinical picture of DVD. Love and Fitzgerald (1984) reported a case that had been followed for more than 5 years—from the age of 2 years, 5 months to 7 years, 9 months—at a community hearing and speech center. Hall et al. (1990) described a suspected DVD case for a total of 11 years, beginning at age 7. In the former case, the longitudinal observation allowed the speech-language pathologists to come to a final diagnosis of DVD. In the latter case, the long-time observation allowed the authors to assess the effectiveness over several years of a new therapeutic procedure—the use of a palatal lift prosthesis. They were able to evaluate the course of improvement in hypernasality articulation and language over long periods of palatal lift prosthesis use and speech therapy.

Second, the case study format allows intensive study of a critical area of performance relating to DVD. Grunwell and Yavas (1988) studied extensively the phonetic and phonologic abilities of a 9-year-old boy with disordered phonologic development who was suspected of a neurologic motor programming disorder. The results of the careful phonetic analysis revealed a productive phonology exhibiting a well-developed segmental phonetic repertoire in conjunction with extremely restricted phonetic structures. The authors argue that the severe constraints upon combining and sequencing the segments of the phonetic system were directly caused by the motor programming disability, which in turn restricted phonetic potential, eventually creating a constrained and disordered phonologic system.

Third, the case study format may provide new information in the important area of clinical management of DVD. The Hall et al. (1990) study of the use of a palatal lift to improve hypernasality in DVD is the first time this therapeutic technique has been reported in DVD. Although the technique has been extensively used in both adult and child dysarthria, its effectiveness in DVD management has up to now been undetermined.

Fourth, the case study format provides insight into the different clinical patterns of DVD. For the most part, the case study literature primarily reports severe cases of DVD. For instance, Daly et al. (1972) describe a child so dyspraxic that he could hardly speak and who was at first misdiagnosed as mentally retarded, aphasic, or autistic. This type of child with DVD has sometimes been labeled "nonverbal" and most often has been considered a subcategory of childhood or developmental aphasia (Eisenson, 1984). As such, the child with DVD has been considered very uncommon in the total population of childhood communication disorders. Even the DVD child who presents as a severe misarticulating child has been considered rare (Rosen-bek et al., 1974). Some speech-language pathologists who view DVD as a subclass of the population of children with developmental phonologic disability believe there may be greater numbers of children with DVD than was previously assumed (Air & Wood, 1985; Frisch & Handler, 1974; Haynes, 1985), but the claim is not proven. The child severely disabled in speech and language development by dyspraxia may be easier to identify than is the child with DVD who mirrors the child with developmental phonologic disability with multiple misarticulations. More research is needed to distinguish these various subgroups of suspected DVD.

In summary, the single case study approach in DVD has presented rich descriptive evidence of DVD syndromes that go a long way to support the validity of the diagnosis, despite the skepticism voiced about the clinical entity. An example of a case study of one child with severe misarticulation of dyspraxic origin, more fully described in Love and Fitzgerald (1984), was presented in Chapter 1. In addition, the case study approach has been used to present a variety of management techniques for the child with DVD. Careful and detailed case studies, both of the nature and management of DVD, may provide clues for further research that will allow us to better understand DVD and ultimately resolve the controversies surrounding it.

RECENT DEVELOPMENTS

The Iowa and Crary Textbooks

Since the publication of this text, there have been several new contributions to the literature of DVD. In 1993, two major textbooks were published. The first book, which I call the Iowa book because its authors are members of the staff of the University of Iowa, is entitled *Developmental Apraxia of Speech: Theory and Clinical Practice*. Its authors, Penelope K. Hall, Linda S. Jordan, and Donald A. Robin (1993), appear to have had considerable experience with DVD children. The material is straightforward and marshals the facts currently available about the nature and treatment of this controversial disorder.

Having assumed that DVD is primarily a motor speech problem, the authors devote Chapter 3 to theories of motor control and their potential for explaining DVD. After a careful review of six of the current motor theories, the authors conclude that "none of the theories have previously been suggested or yet have been demonstrated to account for DAS" (p. 66). Unfortunately, the book fails to present a section on the neurology of the brain as it relates to DVD, which limits its usefulness as a classroom text. A basic knowledge of the anatomy and physiology of the brain is certainly essential to the understanding of DVD, just as it is to the understanding of any of the motor theories now current. Familial and genetic factors are discussed in Chapter 5, and neurological and psychological symptoms occurring with DVD are documented carefully in Chapter 6. Chapters 7 through 9 are devoted to several aspects of remediation. In brief, the book is an excellent introduction of the complex disorder for the beginning student of neurological speech disorders.

In *Developmental Motor Speech Disorders* (1993), Michael A. Crary, who has been a consistent contributor to DVD for the past several years, presents a fully realized account of his thinking on childhood motor speech disabilities, particularly DVD. Chapter 1 offers historical perspectives and presents a very complete description of *congenital suprabulbar paresis,* which can be easily misdiagnosed as DVD. Crary notes the syndrome, which was first described by the British neurologist C. Worster-Drought (1956), is primarily an upper motor neuron developmental dysarthria that is unaccompanied by the abnormal reflex and paralytic signs seen in the limbs of the typical child with cerebral palsy.

At about the same time the Worster-Drought syndrome was being described, Muriel Morley (1957) reported *acquired articulatory apraxia* in a group of 12 children living in Newcastle-upon-Tyne in Great Britain. Her report brought the concept of DVD to the attention of modern-day speech pathology and neurology (see Love & Webb, 1996, p. 275).

In Chapters 2 and 3, Crary goes on to describe various theories of normal and abnormal brain development and incorporates several current theories of possible maldevelopment and their relation to childhood motor speech disorders. In Chapter 4, he constructs a series of developmental and clinical speech profiles of the child with speech apraxia. Chapter 5 is devoted to specific motor speech performance, including speech gymnastics and speech diadochokinesis as well as to profiles of speech performance exhibiting executive and motor planning skills. The highlight of Chapter 6 is Crary's list of 13 phonologic processes used in the description of children suspected of developmental apraxia of speech. In the next chapter, Chapter 7, Crary discusses language performance in speech dyspraxic children. Chapter 8 is an explanation of Crary's own system of assessment strategies. The book ends with a discussion of intervention strategies.

Crary has given the field a scholarly and readable book on the topic of DVD and has presented some unique approaches to the study of developmental apraxia of speech. His ideas, however, often need further research verification. Furthermore, for a textbook that purports to be a comprehensive discussion of developmental motor speech disorders, the dysarthrias of cerebral palsy and of the lower motor neuron disorders are touched upon only lightly. However, Crary's book is more sophisticated than the Iowa book and thus probably more appealing to the graduate student in training and to the working professional who has had considerable experience with DVD.

The Wisconsin Articles

A third major effort to present a comprehensive picture of DVD appeared in 1997 in a three-article series in a single issue of the *Journal of Speech, Language and Hearing Research* (Shriberg, Aram, & Kwiakowski, 1997). The first article provides an up-to-date review of the currently accepted facts on the nature of DVD. The authors then propose one or more subtypes of DVD, either with varying features or a unitary pathognomic feature. While most investigators have felt that a syndrome composed of a varying set of symptoms must be associated with a widely reported, obvious, and constant physical sign that differentiates the syndrome from all other childhood speech problems (Love, 1992), these authors believe that DVD cannot yet be characterized by a single "pathognomic marker."

Discussing the onset and course of DVD, the authors state that most agree onset occurs early in the developmental speech period but that the upper boundary of that speech period is in doubt as many allophones have not been normalized by adulthood. They go on to say that it is unclear whether normalization of suspected DVD occurs through spontaneous improvement, and they contend that neither late onset of speech nor late normalization of speech can be predicted with any degree of accuracy at this point.

The authors state that gender ratios for developmental phonological items are uncertain, but 2:1 to 3:1 affected males to females are the ratios most often reported, although some investigators have reported higher ratios, thus suggesting an X-linked or X-influenced genetic disorder. Prevalence estimates have ranged from 1 to 1.3% of the population. In contrast, the authors estimate that 5% of preschool children have phonologic disorders of unknown origin. Estimates suggest that DVD has a prevalence rate of 1 to 2% of 1,000 live births, which places it in the category of a low incidence disorder. When compared to children with uncomplicated phonologic speech delay, the frequency of DVD in the population is quite small.

The authors also point out that at least some forms of DVD occur in familial aggregations, which would suggest several modes of genetic transmission. As no phenotype marker has yet been identified, the disorder cannot be studied with the new tools in behavioral or molecular genetics.

After this concise and useful summary of the pertinent facts about the disorder, the authors present several theories of the possible deficit in DVD. Of all the theoretical positions considered, they state that the most popular considers DVD to be a prearticulatory sequencing deficit.

The Research Studies.   Next, the authors present the first portion of their research, which supports the adjective *suspected* in conjunction with DVD, notes the lack of diagnostic markers, and denies the claim that DVD necessarily represents a deficit in linguistic stages. This idea, they maintain, counters the traditional use of the term apraxia.

Articles two and three report the results of the authors' research, which purports to isolate a pathognomic marker that would be useful in diagnosing a child with DVD. The marker in question is determined by perceptual cues alone, ignoring direct study of disturbed motor patterns, which have been considered a feature of dyspraxia for several decades.

The authors' first article provides a comparison of the speech and prosody-voice profiles of 73 children exhibiting speech (phonologic) delay (SD) with the profiles of 14 children with suspected DVD. The article states that the only perceptual feature that separated the two groups was inappropriate stress on the part of the DVD child. One should note that of 14 children suspected of DVD, only 6 actually failed a prosody-voice screening instrument, indicating clear developmental speech apraxia (p. 301).

The third article presents an argument for a subtype of DVD marked by inappropriate stress and reports on an internal cross-validation test of stress as a diagnostic marker for a subtype of DVD. Twenty children with suspected DVD were studied, using a variety of linguistic measures. Data for cross validation of a "stress subtype" of DVD came from a conversational sample of another 19 children suspected of DVD from diverse parts of the country. Although the authors believe they have identified a stress diagnostic marker, they admit their cross-validation research has obvious design limitations, primarily the result of the small sample size of true verbal dyspraxics. In a third study, 52 of the speech samples from 53 children suspected of DVD had inappropriate stress. This frequency of inappropriate stress compared sharply with 10% of 71 eligible samples of conversation from children with speech delay of unknown origin.

Discussion of the Studies.   As the authors discuss the results of their three studies, they generate five hypotheses concerning the meaning of their data for research in DVD. Finally, they draw three conclusions: (1) conversational data indicated phrasal stress was the only linguistic variable that differentiated 52% of these children from age-matched children with speech delay of unknown origin; (2) observations from several sources suggest that the disorder is of neurological origin and genetically transmitted; (3) the stress deficit in DVD occurs within linguistic representational levels of prearticulatory sequencing processes of phonology. There are, the authors note, significant differences between acquired apraxia in adults and their findings in this subtype of DVD, raising the question of whether it is an apraxic motor speech disorder.

Evaluation of the Wisconsin Studies. There is no question that the most critical facts of DVD are well marshaled in the first article, and one is indebted to the authors for clarifying the present state of knowledge about the disorder, particularly in the areas of prevalence and genetics. It is quite clear from the authors' work that despite all the questions a speech-language pathologist faces in making a valid diagnosis, the disorder remains in a low incidence category when compared to speech (phonology) delay of unknown origin.

Indeed, it is surprising that such an uncommon disorder is demanding so much attention in the speech-language disability community; possibly it is intriguing because we lack critical information, because the information we do have is controversial, and because despite these serious issues, the diagnosis of DVD seems valid and appropriate for some children. If one looks closely at the Wisconsin research, however, one begins to question how many aspects of DVD are really explained by the studies and how much the studies resolve the controversies surrounding the disorder.

Waldron (1998) has sharply criticized certain aspects of the Wisconsin research. Charging that the subject selection is flawed, Waldron notes that the first sample of subjects was seen in a previous study of apraxia of speech. She also documents the apparent weakness of the experimental scale (Speech Disorders Classification System) used to classify a child with suspected DVD. She further points out that the one and only criterion for selecting children without DVD was phonologic delay of unknown origin. According to Waldron, the second sample of children also were selected with less than rigorous and consistent criteria, resulting in an ill-defined comparison group.

Waldron also notes that consistency and variability of sound production are not adequately captured in the studies. She complains about the interpretation of selective data in certain figures, ignored data, and the lack of clarity as to whether severity or intelligibility are factors in suggesting differences between younger and older children in displaying a diagnostic marker of DVD. Waldron believes that the data on speech rate is confused, and she notes that the conclusion of suspected DVD is based on only 16 children of varying ages and backgrounds. Finally she asserts that identifying a phrasal stress in only 8 children is hardly a basis for establishing a subtype of DVD. In summary, Waldron believes the research to be too flawed on too many levels to assert that a new form of DVD has been identified.

In response to Waldron, the authors defended their selection process in the three studies by arguing that referrals by experienced clinicians and by several clinical researchers, each using their own inclusion criteria, seemed to be a reliable method of identifying the child with suspected DVD. The criteria, the authors note, were "purposefully unconstrained in order to include in these studies children with the range of features for suspected DAS described in the literature." (Shriberg, Aram, & Kwiatkowski, 1997, p. 961). The authors then point out that the selection process, based on individual criteria, provided them with a very diverse group of subjects from which they identified a possible diagnostic marker, inappropriate stress, as a subclass of DVD.

Whether this diagnostic marker is an indicator of the motor disturbance of apraxia, as introduced into the field of neurology by Hugo Leipman in 1908, is questionable. Certainly the present author believes a one-sided approach is taken in the research. In fact, since respected speech-language pathologists question whether there are ever necessary and sufficient reasons to even postulate a concept of DVD, it seems premature to proclaim a subtype of the condition. Relying on perception alone and interpreting the perceptual data in terms of linguistic theory only may invalidate the results of the study. Indeed, the authors found themselves in the ironic position of having to admit that their diagnostic marker did not identify a true apraxia or motor disturbance (p. 313).

Incorporating current technology into their research design would have allowed the authors to study speech and nonspeech oral movements directly. Smith, Goffman, and Stark (1995) have described the Optotrack, a system that allows recording of the movements or oral structures without any device on the head. A small light emitting disc is placed on the lips, tongue, or jaw, and movement is tracked by cameras with a high degree of accuracy. Digital videoflouroscopy, another current imaging technique, could have provided direct data of motor activity. The technique permits viewing of series speech or nonspeech oral movement without fear of excessive radiation (B. Shack, M.D., personal communication, October 1998). This technique is used widely by craniofacial anomaly centers.

SUMMARY

Developmental verbal dyspraxia (DVD) is usually considered a motor speech disorder characterized by awkward groping movements of the articulators and an inability to consistently position the articulators for speech. This inability to execute voluntarily the appropriate movements for articulation must be, in the absence of paralysis and weakness or incoordination, caused by pyramidal, basal ganglia, or cerebellar dysfunction. In verbal dyspraxia, movements unavailable in speech may be observed in automatic nonspeaking acts. A related concept is oral or buccofacial apraxia. Oral nonspeech apraxia usually is defined as an inability to perform oral movements on command with the muscles of the larynx, pharynx, tongue, cheeks, and lips, although more automatic movements of muscles may be retained in such activities as biting, chewing, and swallowing.

The concept of developmental verbal dyspraxia is controversial on several levels. It has been thought of as analogous to the adult condition of speech apraxia seen most frequently in Broca's aphasia, but the lateralized and focal brain lesions that are traditional in the adult with speech apraxia do not fit the neurologic findings in children. If there are brain anatomy correlates in childhood verbal dyspraxia, they generally are most likely to be a structurally normal-appearing brain with the possible exception of some minor developmental anomalies. Genetic factors may play a role in etiology in some cases.

A strong argument can be made that the critical physical sign of the disorder is poor motor programming in speech movements and/or oral movements. It is recommended that the presence of an oral apraxia be considered as part of an operational definition of developmental verbal dyspraxia. The better designed studies in the field have included careful oral apraxia testing in their protocols. Motor programming disorders appear to be a more reliable sign of the disorder than do specific patterns of phonologic errors, language impairment, minor neurologic signs, or poor response to therapy. Other deficits may accompany the speech and oral motor programming problems, but no set of signs and symptoms is universally accepted as a dyspraxic cluster.

Several attempts have been made to isolate developmental verbal dyspraxic subgroups from the larger population of children with functional articulation disorders. Much effort has been expended on defining unique phonologic error patterns, but results are conflicting largely because of limited research designs. Many research studies of DVD are flawed by the lack of an equated control group without suspected dyspraxia. Controlled studies using equated groups have failed to replicate phonologic and other characteristics said to be typical of DVD in misarticulating children. In the face of equivocal group findings, investigators have turned to single case studies as an alternate research strategy to document in a detailed manner the natural history of the disorder. Innovative and carefully designed research is desperately needed if the disorder is to be scientifically described and validated beyond question.

Since the 1992 edition of this book, interest in this controversial, low incidence disorder has remained unabated. Two major textbooks (Hall, Jordan, 1993; Crary, 1993), as well as a major research project consisting of three separate articles (Shriberg, Aram & Kwiatkowski, 1997), have been published.

While several other chapters and articles have appeared, the Crary book, the Iowa book, and the Wisconsin research studies are the most impressive additions to this topic to date. While the Wisconsin articles offer a masterful update of pertinent information, the studies proclaiming inappropriate stress as a diagnostic marker of a subclass of DVD are disappointing, completely dismissing the defining feature of the disorder—the motor disturbance in speech and oral movements.

SUGGESTED READING

Shriberg, L. D., Aram, D. M., & Kwiatkowski, J. (1997). Developmental apraxia of Speech: I. Descriptive and theoretical perspectives. *Journal of Speech, Language and Hearing Research, 40,* 273–285.

This is the best current review of the facts of developmental verbal dyspraxia in the literature of speech-language pathology.

Thompson, C. K. (1988). Articulation disorders in the child with neurogenic pathology. In N. J. Lass, L. V. McReynolds, J. L. Northern, & D. E. Yoder (Eds.), *Handbook of speech-language pathology and audiology* (pp. 548–590). Burlington, Ontario: B. C. Decker.

This chapter is an extensive presentation of the developmental dysarthrias of cerebral palsy and developmental verbal dyspraxia. The section on developmental verbal dyspraxia carefully documents the issues in the controversy about the disorder and presents some positive therapy approaches.

REFERENCES

Air, D., & Wood, A. (1985). Considerations for organic disorders. In P. Newman, N. Creaghead, & W. Second (Eds.), *Assessment and remediation of articulatory and phonological disorders.* Columbus, OH: Merrill.

Aram, D. M., & Nation, J. E. (1982). *Child language disorders.* St Louis, MO: C. V. Mosby.

Bashir, A. S., Grahamjones, F., & Bostwick, R. Y. (1984). A touch-cue method of therapy for developmental verbal apraxia. *Seminars in Speech and Language, 5,* 127–137.

Benson, D. F. (1979). *Aphasia, alexia, and agraphia.* New York: Churchill Livingstone.

Bowman, S. N., Parsons, C. L., & Morris, D. A. (1984). Inconsistency of phonological errors in developmental verbal dyspraxic children as a factor of linguistic task and performance load. *Australian Journal of Human Communication Disorders, 12,* 109–119.

Chappell, G. E. (1973). Childhood verbal apraxia and its treatment. *Journal of Speech and Hearing Disorders, 38,* 362–368.

Cook, T. D., & Campbell, D. T. (1979). *Quasi-experimentation: Design and analysis issues for field settings.* Boston: Houghton Mifflin.

Crary, M. A. (1984). Phonological characteristics of developmental verbal apraxia. *Seminars in Speech and Language, 5,* 71–83.

Crary, M. A. (1993). *Developmental motor speech disorders.* San Diego, CA: Singular Publishing Group.

Daly, D. A., Cantrill, R. P., Cantrill, M. L., & Aman, L. A. (1972). Structuring speech therapy contingencies with an oral apraxic child. *Journal of Speech and Hearing Disorders, 37,* 22–32.

Darwish, H., Pearce, P. S., Gaines, R., & Harasym, P. (1982). The speech programming deficit syndrome. *Annals of Neurology, 12,* 211.

Deputy, P. N. (1984). The need for description in the study of developmental verbal dyspraxia. *Australian Journal of Human Communication Disorders, 12,* 3–13.

DeRenzi, E., Pieczuro, A., & Vignolo, L. A. (1966). Oral apraxia and aphasia. *Cortex, 2,* 749–756.

Edwards, M. (1973). Developmental verbal dyspraxia. *British Journal of Communication Disorders, 8,* 64–70.

Eisenson, J. (1984). *Aphasia and related disorders in children* (2nd ed.). New York: Harper & Row.

Ekelman, B. L., & Aram, D. M. (1984). Spoken syntax in children with developmental verbal dyspraxia. *Seminars in Speech and Language, 5,* 97–110.

Ferry, P. C., Hall, S. M., & Hicks, J. L. (1975). "Dilapidated" speech: Developmental verbal dyspraxia. *Developmental Medicine and Child Neurology, 17,* 749–756.

Frisch, G., & Handler, L. (1974). A neuropsychological investigation of functional disorders of speech articulation. *Journal of Speech and Hearing Research, 17,* 432–445.

Grunwell, P., & Yavas, J. (1988). Phonotactic restrictions in disordered child phonology: A case study. *Clinical Linguistics and Phonetics, 2,* 1–16.

Guyette, T. W., & Diedrich, W. H. (1981). A critical review of developmental apraxia of speech. In N. J. Lass (Ed.), *Speech and language: Advances in basic research and practice* (Vol. 5, pp. 1–48). New York: Academic Press.

Hall, P. K., Hardy, J. C., & LaVelle, W. E. (1990). A child with signs of developmental apraxia of speech with whom a palatal lift prosthesis was used to manage palatal dysfunction. *Journal of Speech and Hearing Disorders, 55,* 454–460.

Hall, P. K., Jordan, L. S., & Robin, D. A. (1993). *Developmental apraxia of speech: Theory and clinical practice.* Austin, TX: Pro-ed.

Harlan, N. T. (1984). Treatment approaches for a young child evidencing developmental verbal apraxia. *Australian Journal of Human Communication Disorders, 12,* 121–127.

Haynes, S. (1985). Developmental apraxia of speech: Symptoms and treatment. In D. F. Johns (Ed.), *Clinical management of neurogenic communication disorders* (2nd ed., pp. 259–266). Boston: Little, Brown.

Helfrich-Miller, K. (1984). Melodic intonation therapy with developmentally apraxic children. *Seminars in Speech and Language, 5,* 119–126.

Horwitz, S. J. (1984). Neurologic findings in developmental verbal apraxia. *Seminars in Speech and Language, 5,* 111–118.

Jaffe, M. B. (1986). Neurological impairment of speech production: Assessment and treatment. In A. Holland & J. M. Costello (Eds.), *Handbook of speech and language disorders* (pp. 157–186). San Diego, CA: College Hill Press.

Kirshner, H. S. (1986). *Behavioral neurology: A practical approach.* New York: Churchill Livingstone.

Klick, S. (1985). Adapted cueing technique for use in treatment of dyspraxia. *Language, Speech, and Hearing Services in Schools, 16,* 256–259.

Lee, L. (1974). *Developmental sentence analysis.* Evanston, IL: Northwestern University Press.

Lewis, B. A. (1990). Familial phonological disorders: Four pedigrees. *Journal of Speech and Hearing Disorders, 55,* 160–170.

Love, R. J. (1992). Developmental verbal dyspraxia. In R. J. Love (Ed.) *Childhood motor speech disability* (pp. 94–111). New York: Macmillan.

Love, R. J., & Fitzgerald, M. (1984). Is the diagnosis of developmental apraxia of speech valid? *Australian Journal of Human Communication Disorders, 12,* 170–178.

Love, R. J., & Webb, W. G. (1996). *Neurology for the speech-language pathologist* (3rd ed.). Boston: Butterworth-Heinemann.

Morley, M. E. (1957). *The development and disorders of speech in childhood* (lst ed.). London: Livingstone.

Morley, M. E. (1972). *The development and disorders of speech in childhood* (3rd ed.). London: Livingstone.

Oyster, C. K., Hanten, W. P., & Llorens, L. A. (1987). *Introduction to research: A guide for the health science professional.* Philadelphia: Lippincott.

Panagos, J. M., & Bobkoff, K. (1984). Beliefs about developmental apraxia of speech. *Australian Journal of Human Communication Disorders, 12,* 39–53.

Parsons, C. L. (1984). A comparison of phonological processes used by developmentally verbal dyspraxic children and non-dyspraxic phonologically impaired children. *Australian Journal of Human Communication Disorders, 12,* 93–107.

Prichard, C. L., Tekieli, M. E., & Kozup, J. M. (1977). Developmental apraxia: Diagnostic considerations. *Journal of Communication Disorders, 12,* 337–348.

Rapin, I. (1988). Disorders of higher cerebral function in preschool children. Part I. *American Journal of Diseases of Children, 142,* 1119–1123.

Rosenbek, J. C., & Wertz, R. T. (1972). A review of 50 cases of developmental apraxia of speech. *Language, Speech, and Hearing Services in Schools, 3,* 23–33.

Rosenbek, J., Hansen, R., Baughman, C. H., & Lemme, J. (1974). Treatment of developmental apraxia of speech: A case study. *Language, Speech, and Hearing Services in Schools, 5,* 13–22.

Shelton, M., & Graves, M. (1985). Use of visual techniques in therapy for developmental apraxia of speech. *Language, Speech, and Hearing Services in Schools, 16,* 129–131.

Shriberg, L. D., Aram, D. A., & Kwiatkowski, J. (1997 a, b, c). *Journal of Speech, Language and Hearing Research, 37,* 273–337.

Shriberg, L. D., Aram, D. M., & Kwiatkowski, J. (1998). Alternate research perspectives: A response to Waldron. *Journal of Speech, Language and Hearing Research, 45,* 960–963.

Smith, A., Goffman, L., & Stark, R. E. (1995). Speech motor development. *Seminars in Speech and Language, 16,* 87–95.

Thompson, C. K. (1988). Articulation disorders in the child with neurogenic pathology. In N. J. Lass, J. L. Northern, & D. E. Yoder (Eds.), *Handbook of speech-language pathology and audiology* (pp. 548–590). Burlington, Ontario: B. C. Decker.

Waldron, C. M. (1998). Comments regarding the investigation of developmental apraxia of speech: Response to Shriberg, Aram and Kwiatkowski. *Journal of Speech, Language and Hearing Research, 41,* 958–960.

Weiner, P. S. (1969). The perceptual level functioning of dysphasic children. *Cortex, 5,* 440–457.

Wertz, R. T., LaPointe, L., & Rosenbek, J. C. (1984). *Apraxia of speech in adults: The disorder and its management.* New York: Grune & Stratton.

Williams, R., Ingham, R. J., & Rosenthal, R. (1981). A further analysis for developmental apraxia of speech in children with defective articulation. *Journal of Speech and Hearing Research, 24,* 496–505.

Worster-Drought, C. (1956). Congenital supra bulbar paresis. *The Journal of Laryngology and Otology, 70,* 453–463.

Yoss, K. A., & Darley, F. L. (1974a). Developmental apraxia of speech in children. *Journal of Speech and Hearing Research, 17,* 399–416.

Yoss, K. A., & Darley, F. L. (1974b). Therapy in developmental apraxia of speech. *Language, Speech, and Hearing Services in Schools, 5,* 23–31.

▶ 6

Assessment

*Diagnosis remains the fundamental task . . . because in
last analysis intelligent treatment, guidance and supervi-
sion must rest upon accurate diagnostic appraisal. This is
particularly true of developmental conditions.*
—*ARNOLD GESELL AND*
CATHERINE AMATRUDA, 1941

Introduction to Childhood Dysarthria Assessment
  Plan of Assessment

Oral-Motor Evaluation of the Prespeaking Child
  Assessment through Modified Feeding • Cranial Nerve Format

Clinical Testing for Dysphagia
  Love-Hagerman-Tiami Clinical Dysphagia Examination

Abnormal Oral Reflexes and Deviant Oral-Motor Behavior
  *Common Abnormal Oral Reflexes • Other Oral-Motor Assessment Scales •
  Oral-Sensory Capacities*

Radiologic Examination in the Dysphagic Child
  *Technique of the Examination • Classification of Swallowing Disorders •
  Radiologic Dysphagia Examination in Cerebral Palsy*

Oral-Motor Evaluation of the Speaking Child
  The Robbins-Klee Protocol

Assessment of Speech Production Subsystems in Childhood Dysarthria
  *Respiratory Dysfunction • Laryngeal Dysfunction • Velopharyngeal
  Dysfunction • Articulation Dysfunction • Speech Intelligibility*

Cognitive-Linguistic Assessment
　Assessment Goals • *Neuropsychological-Developmental Assessment*

Developmental Verbal Dyspraxia Assessment
　Current Tests • *Suggested Assessment Battery*

INTRODUCTION TO CHILDHOOD DYSARTHRIA ASSESSMENT

Plan of Assessment

Careful and comprehensive assessment of the infant or child with an obvious or suspected motor speech disability has become unquestionably accepted as an integral part of an effective communication management program. At the very least, the assessment should encompass appraisal of (1) oral motor abilities, including voluntary nonspeech movements, feeding, and dysphagic behavior (clinical and radiologic); primitive oral reflexes; and oral-sensory capacities; (2) speech production subsystems, including respiratory, laryngeal, velopharyngeal, articulatory functions, and speech intelligibility; and (3) cognitive-linguistic functions.

The structure of each assessment varies with the age of the child under evaluation. Jaffe (1986) notes that the Handicapped Children's Early Education Act of 1968 resulted in the establishment of early education programs for neurologically handicapped and developmentally disabled infants, and the Disabilities Education Act of 1975 (PL 94-142) mandated special education for students to the age of 21 years regardless of the severity of the handicap. The result of these two significant legislative acts was to make speech and language services available to groups of children who could benefit from evaluation and treatment of feeding and prespeech behaviors before the onset of the first words. This legislation has highlighted the need for understanding techniques, evaluation, and management of young neurologically impaired children.

ORAL-MOTOR EVALUATION OF THE PRESPEAKING CHILD

It is very common for children with cerebral palsy and other neurologic impairments to come to the pediatrician or child neurologist with an initial complaint of dysphagia (Denhoff, 1976; Fenichel, 1997), but often it is not immediately treated. Parents generally look to the medical community for assistance with the feeding problems of their child, but intervention for the problem is regularly postponed by the physician.

The discipline of speech-language pathology has taken an ambiguous stance toward the evaluation of nonspeech oral movements of prespeaking children with neurologic feeding symptoms. Although pioneer speech-language pathologists (Palmer, 1947; Westlake, 1951) strongly advocated assessment and management of prespeech feeding problems in cerebral palsy as a means of improving oral-motor functioning for later speech, pivotal early research with cerebral-palsied children by Hixon and Hardy (1964) cast doubt on the value of prespeech oral-motor training and negatively influenced many university training programs. On the basis of extensive correlative statistical analysis of intelligibility and speech and nonspeech diadochokinetic rates, Hixon and Hardy (1964) argued that articulation proficiency was strongly correlated with speech diadochokinetic rates rather than with nonspeech diadochokinetic rates. They maintained that nonspeech movements were controlled at different levels in the nervous system and were produced at different rates of movement. This research convinced many speech-language pathologists that evaluation and management of nonspeech oral-motor activities and feeding behaviors were not as effective as direct training of speech in helping the neurologically impaired child. Data gathered by Love, Hagerman, & Tiami (1980) demonstrated that the severity of dysphagia tended to predict degrees of dysarthria, suggesting that nonspeech motor control did affect speech to some degree. Further, Abbs and Rosenbek (1986) argued that comparisons of the several correlations in the 1964 Hixon and Hardy study did not actually support an interpretation of sharp differences between speech and nonspeech motor control in diadochokinetic activities. Moreover, Barlow and Abbs (1984) have demonstrated in their studies of adult spastic dysarthrics that nonspeech control of precise voluntary oral movements parallels the control of precise voluntary movements in speech. This data has led to reassessment of the critical Hixon and Hardy study. In general, reassessment supports the value of assessing and managing the prespeech oral-motor activities of children who are likely to develop childhood dysarthria as their speech emerges.

Assessment through Modified Feeding

Rationale of Evaluation.   Love and Webb (1996) have suggested that chewing and swallowing, as well as neurologic impairment of oral-motor control in infants and young children, can best be evaluated through a technique called **modified feeding,** described by Westlake and Rutherford (1961). The infantile modified feeding examination is carried out by using a small morsel of food (bolus) selectively placed in the oral cavity of the child. The small bolus challenges the child to perform precise movements with the tongue and lips, articulators soon destined to be very important for speech performance.

Both speech and voluntary nonspeech movements appear to be mediated at higher levels in the nervous system, while the reflexive and semi-
voluntary movements of mastication and deglutition are mediated at lower
levels (Abbs & Rosenbek, 1986). A modified feeding examination of oral
muscles, therefore, can only provide limited prediction of the muscle potential for later speech since it assesses functions controlled primarily at levels
of the lower brain stem in infants and very young children. The examination, however, will allow the speech-language pathologist, pediatrician, or
pediatric neurologist to accomplish a gross clinical assessment of the cranial
motor nerves involved in speech and to predict their degree of motor involvement. Since most neurologically impaired infants or very young children are usually unable to comprehend and respond to the physician's adult
cranial nerve examination or the speech-language pathologist's peripheral
oral examination, the technique of modified feeding allows observation of
the bulbar muscle function in a reasonably effective manner.

Chewing and swallowing activities are highly complex motor activities
in the infant's limited repertoire of initial motor behavior and are often
highly sensitive to neurologic dysfunction because of their relatively early
degree of motor integration (Denhoff, 1976). Evidence of dysphagia provides
significant early signs of neurologic damage for the physician (Fenichel,
1997).

Cranial Nerve Format

When the modified feeding technique is used, the demands for precise
movement often trigger abnormal motor signs that will reveal the type of
neurologic dysfunction present in the speech mechanism. Normal children
from 2 to 3 months to 3 years generally respond well to a modified feeding
assessment. Neurologically impaired children beyond 3 years often do well
with this assessment technique as well. The cranial motor nerves in the modified feeding examination are not assessed in the numbered order of the
nerves as they emerge from the brain stem; rather, they are evaluated in the
way in which each nerve functions in chewing and swallowing activities.

The Facial Nerve. The facial nerve (VII) of the child with an oral-motor
problem becomes active when a small morsel of food is placed on the lower
lip in midline. Observations can be made to confirm if lip and lower face
movement are normal or suggest abnormality. Lack of a smiling response between 2 and 4 months may indicate bilateral facial paralysis with poor lip
control. A very sober expression and a limited grin or smile must be evaluated with care to determine if it is a possible neurologic sign suggesting either UMN or LMN disorder. Lack of movement in the lower face but
apparent normal movement in the upper face, particularly in the muscles of

the forehead, usually indicates a bilateral corticobulbar involvement suggestive of spasticity in the child. There is new evidence that facial involvement
in children is spared with a prenatal onset hemiparesis (Lenn & Freinkel,
1989).

An asymmetrical smile with a unilateral flattening of the nasolabial fold
or one side of the face may be a sign of a unilateral paralysis. When accompanied by a lack of homolateral movement in wrinkling the muscles of the
forehead, a unilateral LMN lesion is suspected. This sign sometimes is not as
obvious in the infant and child as in the adult. LMN lesions also may be associated with flaccid facial muscles, including flaccid lips, open mouth posture, and drooling. However, muscle weakness, poor lip seal, and drooling
are also seen in children with spasticity or athetosis.

The Hypoglossal Nerve.   The hypoglossal nerve (XII) controls motor actions of the tongue, and is one of the more important nerves to assess carefully in the modified feeding examination of infants and children. The child
with neurologic impairment is often unable to shape, cup, point, protrude,
retract, lateralize, or elevate the tongue tip in trying to retrieve a bolus of
food from the lips. Lack of vigorous voluntary tongue protrusion is common
in spastic and athetoid children as well as in children with severe LMN disease. In infants with severe neurologic disorder, the tongue may not cup even
during hard crying. Tongue cupping during hard crying can easily be seen
in normal children.

In hemiplegic children with UMN lesions, the tongue will deviate to the
side opposite the suspected lesion. In LMN lesions, the tongue deviates to
the side of the lesion. Tongue atrophy may sometimes be seen in children
with either unilateral or bilateral LMN lesions. Observing unilateral atrophy
of the tongue is relatively simple because half of the tongue with its normal
bulk can be compared with the atrophied half. Bilateral atrophy produces a
small, pointed tongue that appears too small for the oral cavity. Relationships between the presence of atrophy and tongue function in infant chewing and swallowing are not yet clear; how much the loss of muscle bulk adds
to poor motor function in later speech also is unknown.

In spasticity, speed, strength, range, and coordination of the tongue are
often limited in bilateral lesions of the corticobulbar system. In contrast, the
spastic child with a unilateral lesion and an obvious deviated tongue frequently shows little functional impairment. Oral-motor problems are often
more severe immediately after onset but tend to resolve themselves with
time, particularly in unilateral UMN lesions.

In general, the involuntary movements characteristic of basal ganglia
disorders are reflected in the tongue movements of children with dyskinetic
dysarthria. This clearly is true in older children and adults with athetosis.
The infant with congenital hypotonia may evolve into a more classic athetoid

picture when the flaccid tongue that is obvious at first later becomes dominated by involuntary movements.

Excessive tongue thrust, often called an abnormal tongue reflex, is usually observed in children with severe cerebral dysfunction. It is particularly common in athetosis but may be seen in severe spastic quadriplegia on occasion. It can produce an orthodontic problem of open bite and often is associated with severe drooling.

The Trigeminal Nerve. The trigeminal nerve (V) is responsible for biting and chewing motions, and its action can be observed easily in the modified feeding examination. In infancy, the bite and chew pattern has not yet reached full development. Since the infant does not yet have teeth, the bolus of food is merely munched, and there is limited action of the jaw muscles. A mature bite and chew is developed between 2 and 3 years. At this age it is necessary to determine if the neurologically impaired child is able to pulverize a firm bolus of food by the action of the masticatory muscles. It also is important to note if food can be selectively manipulated by the tongue and placed between the teeth for chewing.

In infancy and the first year of life, the tongue is often elevated and a large bolus will be pushed between the anterior hard palate and the blade of the tongue for crushing. Then it is moved directly toward the pharynx. A peristaltic wave of motion of the tongue transports the food into the pharynx. In an older child (2–3 years), a large solid bolus of food can be crushed between the tongue and palate, and then the tongue acts in a whiplike fashion to propel the food laterally between the teeth for grinding and pulverization with vertical, lateral, and rotary jaw movements. This sequence of events confirms the neurologic integrity of the masticatory muscles in older children.

A well-known abnormality in neural control of the jaw muscles is known as an abnormal bite or abnormal jaw or masseter reflex. It is an exaggerated and too-powerful bite response. An abnormal jaw reflex suggests lesions of the UMN above the level of the pons. An abnormal jaw jerk is often seen in neurologically damaged infants and young children and often interferes with normal eating patterns. It may take the form of rapid clonic movements of the lower jaw suggesting the presence of a hyperactive jaw reflex.

The Glossopharyngeal-Vagus Nerves. The vagus and glossopharyngeal nerves (IX–X) are assessed together in the modified feeding examination. The final stage of swallowing, or **deglutition**, occurs after the bolus of food has been well-masticated by jaw movements or crushed between the tongue and hard palate in infants. In this final involuntary swallowing stage, the nasopharynx must be closed; cranial nerves IX and X provide the neural stimulation for elevation of the soft palate and action of the pharyngeal constrictors to accomplish the closure of the velopharynx. A well-known sign of poor velopharyngeal control in infants and children is loss of liquids through the nose.

Unilateral palatal paralysis, either of an UMN or LMN type, may be revealed by asymmetrical action of the palatal arches. With a bilateral disorder, the palate may rest lower than is expected for normal individuals. During velopharyngeal closure, the paralyzed soft palate may be sluggish with either unilateral or bilateral lesions. In mild to moderate UMN damage, the gag reflex may be hyperactive. However, in severe UMN damage, the gag reflex may not be present at all because the degree of motor involvement prohibits muscle action after attempts at reflex stimulation.

The next section provides an alternate technique to modified feeding to assess dysphagic symptoms.

CLINICAL TESTING FOR DYSPHAGIA

Love-Hagerman-Tiami Clinical Dysphagia Examination

Many individuals have asserted that severe and/or persisting dysphagia is likely to be a predictor of childhood dysarthria (Alexander, 1987; Ingram, 1962; Morris & Klien, 1987). It has been difficult to deny or affirm this claim because few dysphagia assessment scales are described in the literature. Love et al. (1980) have produced an experimental clinical dysphagia scale to answer the question of whether dysphagia symptoms or symptoms of abnormal oral reflexes are better predictors of dysarthria in cerebral-palsied individuals. The dysphagia scale, presented in Figure 6-1, assesses five feeding tasks: (1) biting, (2) sucking, (3) swallowing, (4) chewing soft food, and (5) chewing hard food. The literature provides limited data for determining the average times for completion of these tasks in adults or children; however, logical time limits were assigned based on the available data. Each feeding task is tested twice. **Complete failure** is defined as an inability to complete the task either in the initial test or the retest situation.

This particular assessment scale has been helpful to the author in assessing the presence of feeding deficits and in helping to predict if a given child might develop a later dysarthria. Findings on this scale can suggest a need for referral for a more comprehensive radiologic assessment of dysphagia. A more extensive developmental feeding scale has been published by Morris (1982) and has received a good review in the literature (Jaffe, 1986). In comparison, the present scale has brevity and directness in its favor along with established predictive data on a group of 60 cerebral-palsied children with dysarthria.

| | Trial 1 | Trial 2 |
| | (score + or –) | |

1. *Biting:* Breaks completely a piece of Melba toast with movements of upper and lower jaw within 2–3 seconds. (Examiner demonstrates and gives verbal instructions.) _____ _____

2. *Sucking:* Drinks 2 ounces of Kool-aid from a cup through a plastic straw 8.5 mm in diameter. Angle of cup and straw to face is 45 degrees. Task must be completed in 60 seconds. (Examiner gives verbal instructions.) _____ _____

3. *Swallowing:* Drinks and swallows liquid from a cup or straw. Swallow measured either by up-and-down movement of larynx or audible sharp noise during swallow by use of a stethoscope placed over skin lateral to laryngeal prominence. Movement or sound must be present within 45 seconds after drinking liquid. _____ _____

4. *Chewing—soft food:* Lacerates soft food in 15 seconds. Place miniature marshmallows on anterior of tongue. Tell child to chew it up. After 3 or 4 strokes of the mandible, ask child to open mouth to verify that marshmallows are lacerated. _____ _____

5. *Chewing—firm food:* Lacerates firm food in 30 seconds. Place piece of uncooked carrot ½ inch long on the anterior part of tongue. Tell child to chew it up. After 5 or 6 strokes of mandible with rotary jaw action, ask child to open mouth to verify carrot has been well lacerated. _____ _____

Provide two trials of each of the five feeding tasks. Functionally adequate performance in the face of oropharyngeal motor involvement is completion of the five tasks in at least one of two trials of each task. Less than functionally adequate performance in young children is frequently associated with future dysarthria.

FIGURE 6-1   Testing Feeding Performance in Childhood Motor Speech Disabilities

(*Note:* This assessment is best administered at 18 months and beyond. At 18 months, the normal child is no longer dominated by infantile oral reflexes and is beginning to use voluntary feeding behaviors.)

ABNORMAL ORAL REFLEXES AND DEVIANT ORAL-MOTOR BEHAVIOR

Speech-language pathologists who have worked with infants and young children with neurologic damage have been drawn to the study of oral reflex behavior and its abnormalities because of the implications these behaviors may have for infant feeding and speech development. Speech-language pathologists—particularly those trained in neurodevelopmental therapy (NDT) based on the theoretic thinking of Karel and Berta Bobath (1972), who believe cerebral palsy is a manifestation of abnormal reflex behavior—have argued that lack of emergence of oral reflexes will slow the development of normal feeding and may possibly retard the normal course of speech acquisition. They argue that oral reflexes persisting beyond their expected time of disappearance may interfere with the normal course of oropharyngeal development and may disturb later speech production (Sheppard, 1964).

In addition, other speech experts (Shane & Bashir, 1980) have argued that one or more persisting oral reflexes in preschool children serve as indicators that speech will develop poorly and be markedly unintelligible and will mark the child as a candidate for use of an augmentative or alternate communication device. Other researchers (Love et al., 1980; Neilson & O'Dwyer, 1981) have questioned whether abnormal oral reflexes predict, or even play a major role in, later dysarthria in cerebral palsy. Even if abnormal oral reflexes play little or no part in the prediction or severity of future dysarthria, it is well-known that abnormal reflexes do impede the development of normal voluntary feeding behavior in some infants and therefore are of considerable interest to speech-language pathologists and occupational therapists who routinely provide therapeutic programs of feeding management. Despite the controversy over the role of abnormal oral reflexes, it is important that speech-language pathologists understand them.

There have been several descriptions in the literature of abnormal infant feeding and deviant oral reflex behavior, but little agreement exists upon a complete listing of reflexes. The descriptions by Workinger (1988) encompass several common abnormal oropharyngeal reflex patterns and reflect a reasonable integration of the literature on abnormal oral reflexes and other deviant oral-motor behavior. Her list is a basis for the following discussion.

Common Abnormal Oral Reflexes

Workinger describes six common oral patterns that may be considered abnormal oral reflexes and/or deviant oral behaviors because they are not part of the typical oropharyngeal maturation of the normal infant. They clearly interfere with normal feeding behavior. (Alexander [1987] provides an even more extensive list of 11 abnormal oral behaviors that are hazardous to infant eating and drinking.) The six abnormal oral movements described by Workinger appear, in part, to be derivatives of the six basic normal oral reflexes of the newborn: (1) rooting, (2) suckling, (3) swallowing, (4) tongue thrusting, (5) biting, and (6) gagging (Love & Webb, 1996).

In the first six months of life, the normal rooting-suckle reflex predominates. Liquids are taken from the nipple or bottle and foods from the spoon by sucking. Later, solids placed on the gums or tongue elicit munching behavior. The lips become more active with maturation. The normal rooting-suckle reflex and biting reflex become quickly integrated but usually disappear by the end of the first six months.

In the second six months, true voluntary sucking emerges as the preferred pattern for obtaining liquid. Suckling behavior, however, still may be seen in taking food from a spoon and during the new experience of drinking from a cup.

The infant's chewing behavior begins as a phasic bite and release pattern. It then progresses to a vertical chew, and it is not until 2 to 3 years of age that a mature rotary chew is achieved. A sustained bite through a solid bolus of food is seen at about 10 months of age.

Tongue lateralization accompanies the maturation of chewing behavior. At approximately 7 months of age, a gross rolling lateralization of the tongue is present. With time this develops into a more mature side-to-side movement.

The six abnormal reflex patterns described by Workinger and seen in children with feeding disorders are (1) jaw thrust, (2) tongue thrust, (3) lip retraction, (4) tonic bite reaction, (5) tongue retraction, and (6) nasal regurgitation.

Jaw Thrust. The **jaw thrust** is a forceful, downward extension of the mandible. It is likely that the jaw thrust is part of muscle tone changes associated with the postural reflexes of the body. For instance, the abnormal tonic labyrinthine reflex (TLR) response in an infant or child will often be accompanied by extensor hypertonia, which will affect the jaw depressors. The tonic labyrinthine reflex occurs when the head of the infant is extended 45° for a short period of time (Capute, Accardo, Vining, & Rubenstein, 1978). The jaw thrust and general bodily hypertonia are frequently elicited by the presentation and anticipation of food. The jaw thrust can interfere with efficient removal of food or liquid from the spoon, bottle, or cup.

Tongue Thrust. A **tongue thrust**, or tongue reflex, is a forceful protrusion of the tongue from the mouth. The extension phase of the thrust is generally longer than is the retraction phase. The thrust may be highly repetitive. The tongue reflex is often considered part of the normal infant suckle-swallow pattern and is abnormal only after 18 months. It may interfere not only with food and liquid being taken into the mouth but also may prevent adequate transport of food and liquid through the oral cavity and into the pharynx.

Lip Retraction.   In abnormal **lip retraction** the upper lip appears pulled upward, and the lips are retracted as in a smile (Workinger, 1988). This lip posture is said to interfere with appropriate use of the lips in feeding. This abnormal behavior is difficult to explain physiologically since it has been reported that tonic stretch reflexes are uncommon in the lips (Neilson, Andrews, Guitar, & Quinn, 1979). It may be part of a generalized hypertonic reaction in a child with UMN disorder.

Tonic Bite Reaction.   The **tonic bite reaction** is stimulated by touching the jaws, teeth, or gums. In an extreme reaction, the teeth clench strongly for several seconds. This reaction is related to the jaw or masseter reflex that is commonly found in neurologically impaired adults (Love & Webb, 1996). This abnormal reflex frequently frustrates the caregiver when feeding the child, since utensils cannot be manipulated in the oral cavity easily by the feeder.

Tongue Retraction.   **Tongue retraction** is described as a tongue that is pulled into the pharynx with limited range of motion (Workinger, 1988). This reflex, of course, interferes with removal of food from utensils and efficient oral transit. The reaction has not been as widely reported as has the tongue thrust, and its underlying physiology is unknown. One might speculate that it is the result of general bodily hypertonia rather than of oral reflex behaviors mediated at pontine or bulbar levels.

Nasal Regurgitation.   **Nasal regurgitation** is the backward flow of liquid or semidigested food through the nasal cavity. This deviant behavior is associated with abnormal function of the velopharynx. The adequate opening and closing of the velopharynx is dependent upon the neural mechanisms of the gag reflex. Defects in the timing and range of velopharyngeal movements have been documented in almost all types of childhood dysarthria.

Other Oral-Motor Assessment Scales

Several behavioral scales allow assessment of the previously described behaviors and related development. The *Prespeech Assessment Scale* (Morris, 1982), noted earlier, assesses motor development and prespeech behavior below 2 years. Feeding, respiration, phonation, and sound play are evaluated along with various dimensions of gross motor development. Useful profiles comparing normal and abnormal development can be derived. Sheppard (1987) has designed a nonstandardized *Preschool Oral Motor Examination* that emphasizes elicitation of several oral reflexes and other early behaviors. It is global in nature and provides a comprehensive protocol for observing the young child with abnormal motor patterns. Mysak (1987) has presented a nonstandardized scale, titled *Evaluation of Basic and Early Skilled Speech Movements.* Derived from earlier work (Mysak, 1980), it is based on his neuroevolutionary theory of cerebral palsy. It goes well beyond assessment of oral and speech behaviors, examining back, elbow, sitting, standing, and hand postures. Interpretation guidelines for findings are not given. These three scales provide information similar to that derived from modified feeding testing, the clinical dysphagia examination, and assessment of abnormal oral reflexes.

Oral-Sensory Capacities

Child dysarthria experts (Hardy, 1983; Stark, 1985) generally maintain that dysarthria is a sensorimotor problem, rather than just a motor problem. In the 1960s, a number of studies documented that oral-sensory defects play a role in the speech performance of cerebral-palsied children. Both oral-tactile sensitivity and oral-stereognostic abilities, particularly in spastic hemiplegic children, were found to be impaired.

Tactile sensitivity is most often measured by assessing **two-point discrimination** using an esthesiometer in the speech-science laboratory. The esthesiometer is not easily employed in the clinical situation, and there has not been widespread use of the instrument with populations of dysarthric children. Thus, the magnitude and the effect of sensory loss in the tongue and other articulators has not been well documented in many subgroups of dysarthric children.

Oral-stereognostic testing is another laboratory procedure used to test the loss of oral-sensory capacities. **Stereognosis** is the ability to recognize three-dimensional forms through the senses. This capacity has been tested orally by placing a series of small acrylic forms representing geometric shapes into the mouth of a child without his or her knowledge of the shapes. Lack of recognition of a shape is said to indicate oral-stereognostic impairment. Results of the research on speech-disordered children has been equivocal. In most cases, the ability to recognize shapes in the oral cavity seems to have little or no relation to speech performance. In fact, in one study, a spastic quadriplegic person who demonstrated poor oral two-point discrimination, poor oral form recognition, and an inability to report his tongue position performed acceptably on articulation tests (Love & Webb, 1996).

Clinical neurologists routinely have employed clinical tests of tactile sensitivity to assess possible sensory loss in neurologic impairment. To test sensory loss of the face, neurologists over the years have asked patients to close their eyes and recognize when and where a wisp of cotton touches their faces. Clinically, probe sticks sometimes have been used to attempt to assess sensory capacities of the oral area of cerebral-palsied children with dys-arthria. The child is asked to identify when and where a probe stick is touch-ing the orofacial area.

Caution must be urged when attempting to interpret these relatively crude clinical tests as evidence of somesthetic impairment. Evidence of im-pairment apparently does not mean that there will be a significant negative effect on speech in all cases (Hardy, 1983). The tests are not in widespread use in speech-language pathology because of equivocal findings and the dif-ficulty in interpretation.

RADIOLOGIC EXAMINATION IN THE DYSPHAGIC CHILD

The modified feeding examination, testing of specific feeding tasks, assess-ment of abnormal oral reflexes, and possible oral-sensory assessment have long been considered a part of the routine clinical examination of the dysarthric child. Over the past decade, however, there has been a growing interest in the problem of dysphagia in children and adults. Fenichel (1997) indicates that dysphagia is a significant problem in pediatric medicine. The need for a more revealing, objective, instrumental technique of assessment became apparent because of the frequency with which the problem occurs in children. Radiologic techniques, specifically videofluoroscopy, have become the procedure of choice for evaluating the pediatric patient with a swallow-ing problem (Tuchman, 1989). Videoflouroscopy is a widely available as-sessment and provides the best means for visualizing the oral, pharyngeal, and esophageal anatomy. The technique documents the presence of aspira-tion (sucking of foreign material into the lungs); provides evidence of oral and pharyngeal incoordination; yields information on what characteristics of the bolus of food are swallow-safe in terms of size and consistency; and in-dicates if a child aspirates silently and should be considered a candidate for nonoral feeding (Tuchman, 1989).

Technique of the Examination

The videofluoroscopic examination often begins with scout films of the chest and neck. The swallowing act itself is generally recorded in lateral view and, if possible, in a posterior-anterior projection. The information derived from the modified feeding examination, clinical dysphagia testing, and oral reflex examination, completed by the speech-language pathologist before video-fluoroscopy, may be helpful to the radiologist. For instance, lack of a gag re-flex is considered a contraindication for normal swallow, and a hyperactive gag is considered a sign that there will be significant feeding difficulties (Tuchman, 1989).

Often, withholding a meal prior to the videofluoroscope examination encourages an infant or small child to drink barium more easily. The child is examined, when possible, in the position in which he commonly eats; infants are usually supine and children in a sitting position. Special orthopedic chairs are employed if necessary, and specialized feeding methods and devices for children with specific handicaps may be used during videofluoroscopy (Kramer, 1989).

It should be noted at this point that radiologic dysphagia examination is a relatively new area of practice in speech-language pathology. Considerable experience and training are necessary to perform and correctly interpret videofluoroscopy in dysphagic children. Speech-language pathologists must engage in specialized training to achieve the necessary competence to serve on the dysphagia team and to understand the legal ramifications of this type of dysphagia evaluation. Workshops and textbooks, however, are readily available for those who wish to engage in this newer aspect of speech-language pathology.

Classification of Swallowing Disorders

Swallowing disorders are revealed on videofluoroscopic examination as isolated abnormalities or multiple abnormalities. Kramer (1989) has found it useful to categorize abnormalities in terms of where they occur in the swallowing sequence. As shown in Table 6-1, swallowing abnormalities occur in the oral, pharyngeal, and/or esophageal stages or as global abnormalities.

Radiologic Dysphagia Examination in Cerebral Palsy

Christensen (1989) indicates that the group of children presenting the largest and most difficult challenge to the pediatric dysphagia team are those with cerebral palsy and associated neurogenic feeding disorder. Love et al. (1980) have reported that in their sample of 60 subjects, as many as 40% of the individuals with cerebral palsy had abnormalities in at least one dysphagia task. Christensen asserts that those who show any dysphagic signs require radiologic examination.

The young cerebral-palsied population often demonstrates recurrent aspiration with secondary infection and injury to the developing lung. Moreover, the dysphagic problems in cerebral palsy may lead to inadequate fluid and calorie intake, which results in protein-calorie malnutrition and associated problems. Cerebral-palsied children are also at high risk for gastroesophageal reflux and associated esophagitis, causing painful swallowing.

The pediatric dysphagia team for a child with a suspected or known motor speech disability may vary depending upon the expertise of those involved, but in addition to the speech-language pathologist and radiologist, pediatricians, gastroenterologists, nutritionists, occupational therapists, and pediatric nurses are usually considered likely candidates for the team.

TABLE 6-1   Radiologic Swallowing Abnormalities

Oral Phase

Deficient suckling
Refusal of oral feeding
Failure to develop more mature feeding modes
Oral motor dysfunction
Tongue abnormality
Premature leak into pharynx

Pharyngeal Phase

Delayed onset of pharyngeal swallow
Abnormal soft palate function
Nasopharyngeal reflux
Pharyngeal contraction/emptying deficit
Laryngeal penetration
Cricopharyngeal sphincter abnormality

Esophageal Phase

Secondary aspiration
Esophageal abnormality: anatomical or functional
Gastroesophageal reflux

Incoordination

Source: Kramer, S. S. (1989). Radiologic examination of the swallowing impaired child. *Dysphagia, 3,* 117–125. Reprinted with permission.

ORAL-MOTOR EVALUATION OF THE SPEAKING CHILD

The Robbins-Klee Protocol

Many young children with childhood dysarthria speak with some degree of intelligibility and comprehend directions sufficiently well to perform a systematic assessment of their oral and motor speech abilities. Few tests for children are available to assess these skills accurately. In the past, if the speech-language pathologist wished to assess these abilities with a formal and systematized examination, he or she was forced to rely on the traditional neurologic cranial nerve examination, which is without normative data (Love & Webb, 1996) or on the available motor speech examinations designed by speech-language pathologists for adults (Dworkin & Culatta, 1980; Enderby, 1983; Vitali, 1986).

Robbins and Klee (1987) have developed a motor speech examination for children that recognizes the maturational aspects of the nervous system and provides normative data on children. As seen in Table 6-2, the test consists of 86 items that assess the structure and function of the vocal tract from lips to respiration-laryngeal complex. Both speech and nonspeech aspects are assessed. Normative data is presented on physically normal children for each of nine 6-month intervals from 2 years, 6 months to 6 years, 6 months. Mean and standard deviations are reported for alternate motion rates in syllables and words, and data on maximum phonation is reported for each age interval. A cranial motor nerve format is used to organize the information on structure and function, permitting differential diagnosis of speech production subsystems. In brief, it appears that the *Robbins-Klee Oral and Speech Motor Control Protocol* will provide more accurate and standardized assessment of the oropharyngeal mechanism in childhood dysarthrics and suspected developmental verbal dyspraxics than do other tests now available.

ASSESSMENT OF SPEECH PRODUCTION SUBSYSTEMS IN CHILDHOOD DYSARTHRIA

Experts in motor speech disability (Hardy, 1983; Netsell, Lotz, & Barlow, 1989; Stark, 1985; Thompson, 1988) have suggested that a careful assessment of the physiologic subsystems involved in speaking is important for understanding the dynamics of the individual dysarthric case with its unique variations. Thompson points out that two approaches to subsystem analysis currently are available: instrumental evaluation methods and perceptual analysis methods. The work of Netsell et al. (1989) and Lotz and Netsell (1989) exemplify current instrumental approaches. These approaches, however, are not always available to all speech-language pathologists who deal with childhood dysarthrics, and the majority of clinicians will no doubt rely on perceptual analysis to assess the subsystems of respiration, phonation, resonance, and articulation of children (Darley, Aronson, & Brown, 1975). As Thompson (1988) indicates, it is difficult if not impossible, when using subjective perceptual analysis, to assess separately certain subsystems of speech production. Many of the speech tasks used in a subsystem analysis of dysarthria involve more than one speech subsystem. Another critical point made by Thompson is that subsystem analysis is often highly subjective and errors in judging abnormalities are common. Interjudge reliability in assessing the complex components of dysarthria is not high.

The solution to these problems is, of course, better training of clinicians in perceptual analysis with neurologic speech disorders. Often, time is not set aside in university training programs to train reliability of perceptual judgment of dysarthric speech, and speech pathologists are unsure of their

TABLE 6-2   Robbins-Klee Oral and Speech Motor Control Protocol for Young Children

Lips (CN VII)
Structure at rest:
1. Symmetry
2. Relationship (open vs. closed)
Oral function:
3. Rounding
4. Protrusion (blowing)
5. Retraction
6. Alternate pucker/smile
7. Bite lower lip
8. Lip seal
9. Puff cheeks
10. Open-close lips
Speech function:
11. Rounding /ɔʊ:/
12. Protrusion /u:/
13. Retraction /i:/
14. Alternate /u/, /i:/
15. Bite lower lip /f/
16. Open-close lips /mʌ/
Mandible (CN V)
Structure at rest:
17. Symmetry
18. Occlusion
19. Size (re: facial features)
Oral function:
20. Excursion (click teeth 5×)
Maxilla
Structure at rest:
21. Symmetry
22. Size
Teeth
23. Decay
24. Alignment
25. Gaps
26. Missing
27. Occlusion (re: maxillary teeth)
Tongue (CN XII)
Structure at rest:
28. Symmetry
29. Carriage
30. Fasciculations
31. Furrowing
32. Atrophy
33. Hypertrophy
Oral function:
34. Protrusion
35. Elevation to alveolar ridge
36. Anterior-posterior sweep
37. Interdental
Speech function:
38. Elevation to alveolar ridge:
    /n/, /t/, or /l/
39. Touch lateral edges of tongue
    to teeth: /s/ or /ʃ/
40. Interdental /θ/

41. Posterior tongue to palate:
    /k/ or /g/
Velopharynx (CN X)
Structure at rest:
42. Symmetry
43. Uvula
44. Tonsils
45. Vault height
46. Palatal juncture (palpate)
Oral function:
47. Blow on cold mirror
48. Suck through straw
Speech function:
49. /a:/
50. /ha.ha.ha/
Larynx-Respiration (CN X)
Structure at rest:
51. Posture during quiet breathing
Oral function:
52. Cough, laugh, or cry
Speech function:
81. Maximum phonation time
    (in seconds): /a:/
53. Pitch variation
54. Loudness variation
55. /ha.ha.ha/
Coordinated speech movements
56. (82)[a] /pʌ/ repetitions
57. (83)[a] /tʌ/ repetitions
58. (84)[a] /kʌ/ repetitions
59. (85)[a] /pərəkə/ repetitions
60. (86)[a] *patticake* repetitions
61. you
62. top
63. beef
64. fume
65. cowboy
66. band-aid
67. half time
68. banana
69. kitty cat
70. puppy dog
71. communicate
72. 1950
73. potato head
74. Winnie the Pooh
Speech sample
Prosody:
75. Rate
76. Intonation
Voice:
77. Pitch
78. Loudness
79. Quality
80. Nasal resonance

[a]Items 56–60 are scored for articulatory accuracy, and Items 82–86 for mean number of repetitions per second over 3 s.

skills in this area when working with dysarthric children. However, the following presents a series of simple tasks to evaluate various aspects of speech in dysarthric children that do not rely heavily on instrument methods and involve limited perceptual analysis.

Respiratory Dysfunction

Hardy (1983), in making suggestions on assessment procedures for the speech-language pathologist who does not have access to instrumental techniques, indicates that a precise measurement of the severity of the respiratory function of a given dysarthric child need not be a primary goal because it is highly likely that some respiratory problems are present in most children. Rather, the more important goal is to determine how much the respiratory problem affects speech performance and what limitations it imposes on the speaker for improving his or her speech.

Several simple tasks will provide the speech-language pathologist with a reasonable clinical impression of the breath-control characteristics that determine the quality of the child's usual speech performance. It is important to remember when assessing any of these simple tasks that the respiratory and phonatory systems are interlocked. It is sometimes very difficult to separate the effect of one system from the other in terms of final speech output.

Prolongation of a Neutral Vowel. Prolonged phonation time has long been used as a test of breath support in dysarthric speech. Usually the effort has been timed so that comparisons may be made with available data to determine if the child's ability is seriously deficient for age. Two types of phonation time should be obtained: (a) routine phonation time and (b) maximum-effort phonation time. Comparison of the two times will provide an estimate of what expiratory reserve the child possesses when phonation is produced at relatively high levels of breath support for speech. The duration of prolonged phonation under routine and maximum conditions reveals the child's ability to use the respiratory system to drive the vocal tract under various conditions as well as the ability of the laryngeal system to modify the airstream (Hardy, 1983). Vowel prolongation is usually one of the easiest respiratory tasks for the dysarthric child to perform since the physiologic demands are not as great as in a speaking act in which there are a variety of phonetic contexts with rapidly changing motor gestures.

Counting from One to Ten. Hardy (1983) suggests counting as a good speaking task to test the child's ability to provide breath for a syllable train. The performance should be elicited under two sets of directions: (a) "Count for me until I tell you to stop," and (b) "Take a deep breath and count as long as you can." The first direction elicits routine performance and will allow the speech-language pathologist to assess approximately how many syllables may be uttered on a breath group. The second direction will test the child's respiratory capacities for speaking at high levels of lung volume.

Comparing Voiced CV Repetitions with Voiceless CV Repetitions.   The child who has difficulty in prolonging a vowel is very likely to display difficulty in producing voiced and voiceless CV repetitions (Hardy, 1983). The mean number of syllables produced per second for voiced and voiceless CV repetitions should be calculated so that comparisons can be made between these two speech tasks (Thompson, 1988). Generally, voiced CV syllables are easier to produce than are voiceless CV syllables, and counted morphemes are more difficult than vowel prolongation in voiced/voiceless tasks.

Producing Contextual Speech in Reading or Conversation.   This task of producing contextual speech was used by Darley et al. (1975), without measurements, in their assessment of adult dysarthrics. Thompson (1988) suggests that a significant measure to obtain for contextual speech is mean length of utterance per inhalation. This may be compared with mean length of utterance per inhalation for the counting task. Comparison of these two measures will reveal how demands of length and complexity of utterance are affected by respiratory limitations.

Inspiring and Expiring of a Deep Breath.   The ability to increase lung volume and to control expired air serves as a test of the capacity of the respiratory system without confounding respiration by vocal tasks. Timing of the inspiratory and the expiratory phase is useful because the ability to increase the inspiratory lung volume before an utterance generally increases the length of the expired breath group, and more syllables can be uttered in the breath group. This improves speech prosody (Hardy, 1983).

Finally, a series of observations should be made during the examination to determine the type of respiratory impairment. Short utterances with audible or visible inhalations between each utterance, slowing of speech over time, and strained vocal quality at the end of phrases are often heard; these are common signs of poor respiratory function. In addition, reduced syllable repetitions, decreased overall rate, and uncontrolled exhalation usually are significant signs of impaired respiratory control.

In young children, direct physical examination of the thorax may be helpful in understanding the dynamics of abnormal breathing. Early literature (McDonald & Chance, 1964; Westlake & Rutherford, 1961) has suggested that rapid infantile breathing rates often persist in the neurologically damaged child and interrupt the development of a longer exhalation phase in the inhalation/exhalation cycle. Rates of inhalation more than 30 times per minute generally compromise breath control for speech (McDonald &

Chance, 1964). The result may be shallow inhalations and short exhalations as well as interruptions in the ongoing vocalizations of the child. Tasks requiring loudness variations that are unsuccessfully accomplished are also signs of poor respiratory control. A consistently soft or breathy voice may have its basis in poor respiratory support; similar symptoms may also arise from poor valving at the velopharynx and/or lips in some dysarthric children.

Laryngeal Dysfunction

As already noted, limited research is available on laryngeal dysfunction in dysarthric children. However, the studies of phonatory symptoms in adult dysarthrics make some assumptions fairly reliable. The five vocal tasks previously suggested for testing respiratory dysfunction can also provide data for assessing phonatory problems. The interdependence of the respiratory and laryngeal systems makes this feasible. Hardy (1983) observes that the perceptual quality of the vocal tone during prolongation of a neutral vowel may be the best sign of dysfunction of the intrinsic laryngeal muscles. The neutral vowel precludes abnormal adjustments of tongue positioning because of hypertonicity in the tongue and/or the muscles of the neck, so prolongation of a neutral vowel is a relatively uncontaminated test of laryngeal control.

Obvious differences between the duration of voice CV repetitions and voiceless CV repetitions point to a problem in abduction and adduction of the vocal folds. An additional test used by Westlake and Rutherford (1961) will provide confirmatory evidence for this hypothesis: When a child is asked to imitate a machine gun and say "ah-ah-ah-ah-ah" as fast as he or she can, the resulting sound may be slow, weak, and breathy, or slow and strained. This test assesses rapidity of adduction and abduction of the vocal folds. Further, Westlake and Rutherford note that vocal fold adduction seems to be associated with extensor patterns, and the child with hypotonic muscles, as in some athetoids, may extend the trunk and neck, apparently to assist in adduction. Hardy (1983) observes that glottal or strained initiation of phonation may be another sign of a hyperadduction or a hypertension problem of the vocal folds. In contrast, a relatively consistent breathy initiation generally points to a hypofunctioning problem in laryngeal muscles.

Laryngeal dysfunction can also be diagnosed from reduced pitch and loudness ranges, but the speech-language pathologist must remember that respiratory factors also play a role in loudness and pitch changes. Low pitches may suggest weakness of the vocal folds with a reduced degree of longitudinal tension. This type of weakness is common in childhood dysarthrias with LMN disorders.

Hoarse, harsh, or struggle-strained qualities are commonly heard in spastic adults and, to a lesser degree, are present in children. It has been stated (Thompson, 1988) that fluctuating vocal patterns with sudden uncontrolled variation, phonatory breaks, and tremor are typical of athetoid dyskinesias, but the study by Meyer (1983) does not confirm this. Her work showed very few differences in vocal performance between spastic and dyskinetic children. More research is needed to verify or deny perceptual differences in vocal performance between spastic and athetoid children.

Velopharyngeal Dysfunction

The work of Netsell (1969), as noted earlier, identified a series of several patterns of velopharyngeal dysfunction present in children with the childhood dysarthrias of cerebral palsy. His research, along with the later studies of velopharyngeal dysfunction in dysarthria, suggested that hypernasality and articulation problems resulting from inadequate function of the palatopharyngeal muscles may have very serious consequences on speech intelligibility in dysarthria.

Several tasks can be used to identify inadequate velopharyngeal functioning clinically. Hypernasality and audible nasal omission are key signs of possible velopharyngeal dysfunction in the following tasks:

1. Prolonging of the voiceless continuant /s/. It is well known that adequate production of this phoneme requires a very firm velopharyngeal seal, and inability to achieve that seal or maintain it over time is suggestive of velopharyngeal problems.
2. Counting from one to ten. This sequence of morphemes contains an adequate compliment of fricatives, affricatives, and plosives to test for palatopharyngeal problems. Fricatives, affricatives, and plosives require relatively high levels of intraoral breath pressure and are sensitive to velopharyngeal dysfunction. Caution must be exercised in interpreting results suggestive of velopharyngeal incompetence because misarticulation may also be due, at least in part, to motor involvement of the lips and tongue rather than to velopharyngeal inadequacy. Hardy (1983, p. 129) has given details of expected deviations from normal in terms of hypernasality and articulation when velopharyngeal dysfunction is suspected in the dysarthric child.
3. Testing for consistent visual emission of nasal air during counting or other speech attempts. By placing a cooled dental mirror or other type of emission-sensitive mirror under the nostrils, air emission can be visualized. Fogging of the mirror during production of the nonnasal sounds is suggestive of possible emission problems.

These techniques yield only indirect information about the adequacy of velopharyngeal function. If the problems resulting from dysfunction of the velopharynx are a major hazard to speech intelligibility, assessment by radiologic means should be considered. Videofluoroscopic examination of the velopharynx has become a routine radiologic procedure and can be used with the dysarthric as well as the cleft palate child. Although radiologic assessment of velopharyngeal function in childhood dysarthria may not be as frequent in the radiologist's practice as are cases of craniofacial anomalies, cleft palate team members are currently beginning to see more dysarthric patients, and their expertise in the area of assessing velopharyngeal function in dysarthria is increasing.

Articulation Dysfunction

Articulation Tests.   Speech-language pathologists generally have at their disposal a full range of commercially available materials to assess articulation in childhood dysarthria. It has been routine to assess articulation with single-word articulation tests at the onset of the evaluation. In a basic articulation battery, however, it is advisable to include tests that also provide sentence testing and phonologic processes assessment. Motor complexity in sentence production usually is increased over single words, and the results of sentence testing may provide a clearer picture of what problems the motor-impaired child faces in motor control for phonetic production. Thoughtful selection of test materials will make the analysis of patterns of articulation errors easier and more revealing. We have used two tests frequently: The *Fisher-Logemann Test of Articulation Competence* (Fisher & Logemann, 1971) and McDonald's *Screening Deep Test of Articulation* (McDonald, 1968). The Fisher-Logemann test scoring sheet provides an excellent display of errors analyzed by place and manner. Dysarthria is basically a motor problem and is often characterized by more errors of place than of manner (Platt, Andrews, Young, & Quinn, 1980). The Fisher-Logemann test also provides a convenient catalogue of narrow transcription symbols; narrow transcription is helpful in understanding the complex articulation errors in dysarthria (see Chapter 8 for a further discussion).

The *Screening Deep Test of Articulation* provides a sample of a single phoneme in several contexts, many of which reveal errors in sound production when motor complexity of speech production is increased.

Phonotogic Process Analysis.   Phonologic process analysis often yields added information in childhood dysarthria cases. The process analysis will identify modifications and simplifications of phonologic production. Thompson (1988) states that phonologic process errors in the speech of child dysarthrics generally include cluster reduction, final cluster deletion, and stopping. Caution must be used when interpreting errors in terms of phonologic process analysis because, as Stark (1985) observes, the results of any phonologic analysis must be viewed in relation to the limitations imposed by the child's defective motor control system. The speech performance of the dysarthric child, therefore, does not always reflect the child's knowledge of the phonologic system in his or her environment (see Chapter 8).

Instrumental Acoustic Analysis.   Acoustic analysis, on occasion, may be used to supplement listener perceptual judgment in an expanded evaluation of articulation. The 1975 Kent and Netsell study of ataxic dysarthria documented the potency of spectrographic observations as well as cinefluoroscopic evidence of disturbed articulatory movement patterns in dysarthria. The view that videofluoroscopic analysis is highly useful in motor speech research was further buttressed by the cinefluoroscopic study of five athetoids by the same authors (Kent & Netsell, 1978). Studies such as this reveal the constraints on the articulatory patterns that the motor deficit imposes as well as the compensatory articulatory gestures the child employs in his speech production that do not appear with basic articulation testing and perceptual analysis of the dysarthria.

Other Analyses.   On rare occasions the understanding of the disordered articulation may be increased by using EMG recordings which allow detailed study of the timing of articulatory gestures of lip, jaw, and tongue in the utterance of specific syllables. Strain gauge sensors placed on the mandible or tongue may yield precise information of the velocity and force used in articulation.

Speech Intelligibility

It has not been common in clinical or research reports to document intelligibility levels of dysarthric children, but the virtue of the measure is obvious: It is readily understandable to both expert and lay person alike, and its global nature in terms of encompassing all aspects of speech makes it an excellent measure to rate change in speech. Yorkston and Beukelman (1981) have developed an instrument, entitled *Assessment of Intelligibility of Dysarthric Speech*, that allows assessment of word and sentence intelligibility from stimuli that are read or repeated after an examiner. Using this instrument, an examiner can determine the percentage of single words judged intelligible, a score for rate of intelligible speech and unintelligible speech, and a communication efficiency ratio.

A less formal method for assessing just single-word intelligibility has been developed by the same authors, Yorkston and Beukelman (1980). Single-word intelligibility is calculated on 10 written words or on named pictures from a pool of 50 words. The examiner writes down what he or she believes the child has said. Intelligibility then is determined by comparing the examiner's response with the target words.

COGNITIVE-LINGUISTIC ASSESSMENT

Assessment Goals

Since mental retardation and motor impairment coexist in a significant number of neurologically impaired infants and children, it is of some importance to assess cognitive and linguistic skills. Considerable experience with the cerebral-palsied population has convinced most psychologists and speech-language pathologists that the primary goal is not to obtain an IQ or an age-related language score. One of the strengths of the standard intelligence test is to provide reliable prediction of future performance. Standard intelligence tests are able to accomplish this goal in normal populations with good reliability. In neurologically impaired populations, however, the rate of mental growth is often uneven, and standard tests do not yield their usual predictability.

Rather than to obtain a predictive score, formal tests are used generally to assess the current status of the child in terms of cognitive or linguistic strengths and weaknesses with particular emphasis on visual and auditory modalities. Usually each of these modalities is assessed independently of one another. Stark (1985) recommends an information processing approach to assessment. This approach assumes a hypothesized hierarchy of abilities ranging from the association of stimuli to the discrimination of simple stimuli, integration of stimuli into complex wholes, and the ability to derive concepts from perceptual input, as well as integration of concepts with one another. Finally, attention, memory, higher cortical functions, and constructional abilities are assessed.

Neuropsychological-Developmental Assessment

Wilson and Davidovicz (1987) have presented a scheme for the neuropsychological assessment of the cognitive-linguistic abilities of the neurologically impaired child. Their scheme is based on a neuropsychological-developmental model that exemplifies Stark's suggestions for a hierarchical processing approach. The model includes screening of complex behaviors from the *Wechsler Intelligence Scale for Children—Revised* (Wechsler, 1974) or the *Hiskey-Nebraska Test of Learning Aptitude* (Hiskey, 1966). These tests of higher cortical functions are supplemented by selected measures that tap auditory and visual memory, receptive language, fine motor and graphomotor skills, and academic achievement (Table 6-3). This battery of tests is used because at the present there is no one single test that provides for a systematic evaluation of

TABLE 6-3 Subtest Composition of Clinically Specified Factors and Constructs*

Constructs	Factors	Subtests†
Auditory perception	AP1	ITPA Sound Blending
		GFW Sound Mimicry
	AP2	ITPA Auditory Closure
Auditory discrimination	ADQ	GFW Test of Auditory Discrimination—Quiet subtest
	ADN	GFW Test of Auditory Discrimination—Noise subtest
Auditory cognition	AC1	WPPSI Similarities
		ITPA Auditory Association
	AC2	WPPSI Information
		ITPA Auditory Association
	AC3	WPPSI Vocabulary
		WPPSI Comprehension
Auditory memory	AM1	WPPSI Sentences
		McC Verbal Memory 1
	AM2	McC Verbal Memory 2
	AM3	ITPA Auditory Sequential Memory
Retrieval	SR	McC Verbal Fluency
	PR	NCCEA Word Fluency
	VR	Boston Naming Test
Visual discrimination	VD	H-N Picture Identification
		PTI Form Discrimination
Visual spatial	VSp1	WPPSI Block Design
		H-N Block Patterns
	VSp2	McC Puzzle Solving
	VSp3	NCCEA Right-Left Orientation
		McC Right-Left Orientation
Visual cognition	VC1	WPPSI Picture Completion
		ITPA Visual Reception
	VC2	ITPA Visual Association
		H-N Picture Association
		PTI Similarities
	VC3	ITPA Manual Expression
Visual memory	VM1	H-N Visual Attention Span
	VM2	H-N Memory for Color
		ITPA Visual Sequential Memory
	VM3	PTI Immediate Recall
Graphomotor	GrM1	WPPSI Geometric Designs
		McC Draw-A-Design
	GrM2	McC Draw-A-Person
Fine motor	FM	Purdue Pegboard

Source: From Wilson, B. C., Davidovicz, H. M., in *Seminars in Speech and Language* (Vol. 8; 1). New York: Thieme Medical Publishers, Inc., 1987. Reprinted by permission.

*Tests include: Illinois Test of Psycholinguistic Abilities (ITPA); Goldman-Fristoe-Woodcock Test of Auditory Discrimination (GFW); Wechsler Preschool and Primary Scales of Intelligence (WPPSI); McCarthy Scales of Children's Abilities (McC); Hiskey-Nebraska Test of Learning Aptitude (H-N); Pictorial Test of Intelligence (PTI); Neurosensory Center Comprehensive Examination of Aphasia (NCCEA; Children's Norms)

†The list of tests refers to factors and constructs used in profiling preschool children. An alternate set of subtests is used with school-age children and is available on request.

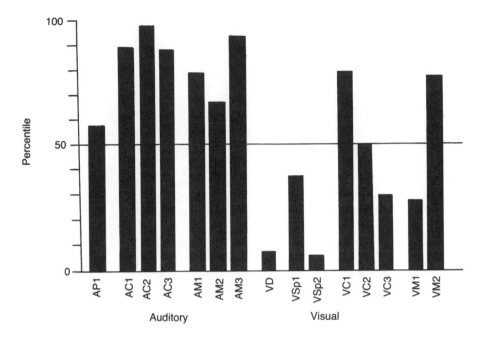

FIGURE 6-2   Profile of a Neurologically Impaired Child
The profile of a 6-year, 3-month-old child with cerebral palsy and left spastic hemiplegia who demonstrates deficits in visual discrimination and in aspects of visual spatial function.

Source: From Wilson, B. C., Davidovicz, H. M., in *Seminars in Speech and Language* (Vol. 8; 1). New York: Thieme Medical Publishers, Inc., 1987. Reprinted by permission.

all critical neuropsychological variables. Since many of the standardized tests used in this battery are based on different metrics, individual test scores are converted into *z* scores and a profile of the child's performance is obtained. This provides a graphic picture of strengths and weaknesses in the neurologically impaired child (Figure 6-2).

Wilson and Davidovicz (1987) argue for flexibility in the evaluation of neurologically impaired children, not only in the selection of test instruments in the battery but also in methods of appraisal. In addition, Stark (1985) indicates that it is crucial to develop valid methods that are nonstandard in cognitive and linguistic testing with motor disabled children. Time limits may have to be extended, repetition of items employed, attention specifically directed, and careful interpretation of isolated skills, or **splinter skills**, must be made. Skills that have not been integrated into usable cognitive functions should not be employed to give an over-optimistic assessment of the child's cognitive-linguistic ability (Stark, 1985).

DEVELOPMENTAL VERBAL
DYSPRAXIA ASSESSMENT

Current Tests

The controversial status of the signs and symptoms of DVD make suggestions for an acceptable battery of diagnostic tests difficult. Only one commercial test has appeared that purports to identify DVD: the *Screening Test for Developmental Apraxia of Speech* (Blakeley, 1980). The test is based on the assumption that a consensus exists in the speech-language pathology community as to a recognized cluster of signs and symptoms that define DVD. The discussion of DVD in Chapter 5 should convince the reader that there is little or no consensus about the defining signs and symptoms of the disorder. Clearly the underlying assumption of the screening test can be challenged.

The Blakely screening test is composed of eight subtests:

    I. Expressive language discrepancy
   II. Vowels and diphthongs
  III. Oral-motor movement
  IV. Verbal sequencing
    V. Articulation
  VI. Motorically complex words
 VII. Transpositions, and
VIII. Prosody.

The test has been submitted to a stinging critical review by Guyette and Diedrich (1983). They found the test lacking in terms of its construction, administration, scoring guidelines, and interpretation. It is reported that the test was developed on a standardization sample of children, ages 4 through 12, who had multiple articulation errors and a broad range of intelligence (Blakeley, 1980). Neither a definition of the types of articulation errors characteristic of the group nor a distribution of errors by age and sex is presented. It is not clear whether the standardization group was drawn randomly from a group of children with presumed functional multiple misarticulations or whether the subjects were suspected DVD children.

Test-retest reliability data are not reported for either the examiner or the children tested. No attempts are made to validate the subtests employed. Scoring guidelines are unclear, and the statistical procedure for determining if a score places a given child in the category of DVD is confusing. The test is labelled a screening test, yet there are no guidelines for further testing or referral for establishing a definitive diagnosis of DVD. This screening test presents serious flaws in terms of adequate design. It clearly does not meet acceptable standards of test construction. Speech-language pathologists familiar with childhood motor speech disability have recommended that it not be used in its present form to screen for DVD (Jaffe, 1986; Thompson, 1988).

Suggested Assessment Battery

Until a well-designed and well-standardized test is developed, speech-language pathologists will be forced to rely on batteries of individually selected tests and clinical judgment for identification of the disorder. Haynes (1985) presents a list of areas of assessment for inclusion in a diagnostic battery, and Love and Fitzgerald (1984) supply a rationale for the logic behind diagnosing a child with suspected DVD as well as list tests they employed with one case. Common areas of assessment employed in both approaches are

1. volitional movements of the oral muscles in isolation and in sequence at both the nonspeech and speech levels.
2. rates of oral diadochokinesis in nonspeech and speech activities.
3. articulatory proficiency of isolated phonemes, polysyllabic words, and connected speech. Love and Fitzgerald also suggest an articulation analysis by place, manner, and error type as well as a judgment of overall speech intelligibility.
4. language testing with standardized language tests.
5. presence or absence of "soft" neurologic signs.

In addition, Haynes recommends assessment of orosensory perception and oral awareness. Love and Fitzgerald recommend ruling out signs of spasticity or flaccidity and the incoordinations of basal ganglia disorder or cerebellar dysfunction; perceptual analysis of vocal characteristics should be made to rule out vocal signs of dysarthria (Darley et al., 1975). Diagnosis is further enhanced if longitudinal assessments are completed or if the suspected DVD case is placed in diagnostic therapy (Love & Fitzgerald, 1984).

SUMMARY

The plan for assessment of children with motor speech disability described in this chapter addresses oral-motor evaluation of (1) the prespeaking child at risk for dysarthria and (2) the child dysarthric speaker. First, a series of procedures is described that primarily apply to the infant and preschool child with oral-motor development disorders. These procedures include a modified feeding examination of the oral muscles that ultimately will be used in speech production. This simple clinical examination, organized in a cranial nerve format, allows observation of an at-risk infant's or child's bulbar muscles as they are used to chew and swallow. The examination provides information that cannot be obtained through the standard cranial nerve examination by the neurologist or the routine peripheral oral examination by the speech-language pathologist. In addition, the modified feeding situation provides an opportunity to observe the development of infantile oral reflexes. Abnormality of these reflexes, in terms of failure to appear at expected ages or persistence of these oral behaviors beyond the time they normally disappear, can be studied by the speech-language pathologist in the modified feeding examination. Although several abnormal oral behaviors have been described in at-risk infants and children, the following were discussed: jaw thrust, tongue thrust, tonic bite reaction, tongue retraction, and nasal regurgitation. When the modified feeding examination indicates a possible serious swallowing disorder, the Love-Hagerman-Tiami Clinical Dysphagia Examination may be employed to determine what swallowing tasks present the most frequent and severe dysphagic symptoms. This assessment scale, designed for children 18 months and older, provides information on five chewing and swallowing tasks. Scores derived from this assessment appear to be better predictors of future dysarthria than are the abnormalities of infantile oral reflexes.

A more revealing dysphagia examination of neurologically impaired children involves radiologic examination of the swallowing function. This examination documents the presence of aspiration and the types and degree of oral-pharyngeal muscle incoordination in different stages of the swallow. Specialized training is necessary for the speech-language pathologist to participate fully on a dysphagia team.

A recent test, the Robbins-Klee Oral and Speech Motor Control Protocol, serves as an excellent standardized assessment instrument for evaluating the young dysarthric speaker. Performance data on physically normal children between the ages of 2 years, 6 months and 6 years, 6 months is reported for this test.

The next step in the evaluation of the dysarthric child speaker is to assess carefully and systematically each of the disturbed physiologic subsystems of speech production. This evaluation includes an assessment of respiratory dysfunction, laryngeal dysfunction, velopharyngeal dysfunction, and articulatory dysfunction, plus an overall assessment of disturbed subsystems by measuring speech intelligibility. A series of subsystem assessment tasks has been drawn from the recent speech literature on child dysarthria. Each of the physiologic subsystems of speech may be assessed without the extensive use of highly technical instrumentation of the speech laboratory.

A comprehensive assessment of the child with dysarthria often demands a neuropsychological assessment to determine the level of cognitive-linguistic functioning. A recently reported neuropsychological developmental test battery by Wilson and Davidovicz, which is well-suited to the assessment of the neurologically impaired child, is recommended.

Finally, the issue of the assessment of the child with a suspected developmental verbal dyspraxia of speech is discussed. Current commercial test batteries for the identification of DVD appear inadequate. Suggestions for assembling a clinical test battery from commonly used diagnostic speech tests are made for the assessment of suspected DVD children.

SUGGESTED READING

Hardy, J. C. (1983). *Cerebral palsy.* Englewood Cliffs, NJ: Prentice-Hall.

Chapter 6 is a judicious approach to assessment of the motor impaired child in the clinical setting. Hardy brings to the task a rich background of experience.

Netsell, R., Lotz, W. K., & Barlow, S. M. (1989). A speech physiology examination for individuals with dysarthria. In K. M. Yorkston & D. R. Beukelman (Eds.), *Recent advances in clinical dysarthria* (pp. 3–37). Boston: Little, Brown.

This chapter presents recent speech science laboratory approaches for assessing childhood dysarthria.

REFERENCES

Abbs, J. H., & Rosenbek, J. C. (1986). Some motor perspectives on apraxia of speech and dysarthria. In J. M. Costello & A. L. Holland (Eds.), *Handbook of speech and language disorders* (pp. 371–407). San Diego: College Hill Press.

Alexander, R. (1987). Oral-motor treatment for infants and young children. *Seminars in Speech and Language, 8,* 87–100.

Barlow, S. M., & Abbs, J. H. (1984). Orofacial fine motor control impairments in congenital spasticity: Evidence against hypertonus, related deficits. *Journal of Neurology, 34,* 145–150.

Blakeley, R. W. (1980). *Screening test for developmental apraxia of speech.* Tigard, OR: C C Publications.

Bobath, K., & Bobath, B. (1972). Cerebral palsy. In P. H. Pearson & C. E. Williams (Eds.), *Physical therapy services in the developmental disabilities.* Springfield, IL: Charles C. Thomas.

Capute, A. J., Accardo, P., Vining, E. P. G., & Rubenstein, J. E. (1978). *Primitive reflex profile.* Baltimore: University Park Press.

Christensen, J. R. (1989). Developmental approach to pediatric neurogenic dysphagia. *Dysphagia, 3,* 131–134.

Darley, F. L., Aronson, A. E., & Brown, J. R. (1975). *Motor speech disorders.* Philadelphia: W. B. Saunders.

Denhoff, E. (1976). Medical aspects. In W. M. Cruickshank (Ed.), *Cerebral palsy: A developmental disability* (3rd rev. ed.) (pp. 31–71). Syracuse, NY: Syracuse University Press.

Dworkin, J., & Culatta, R. (1980). *Dworkin-Culatta Oral Mechanism Examination.* Nicholasville, KY: Edgewood Press.

Enderby, P. (1983). *Frenchay Dysarthria Assessment.* San Diego, CA: College Hill Press.

Fenichel, G. M. (1997). *Clinical pediatric neurology* (3rd ed.). Philadelphia: W. B. Saunders.

Fisher, H. B., & Logemann, J. A. (1971). *Fisher-Logemann Test of Articulation Competence.* Boston: Houghton Mifflin.

Gesell, A. L., & Aramatruda, C. S. (1941). *Developmental diagnosis: Normal and abnormal development.* New York: Paul B. Hoeber.

Guyette, T. W., & Diedrich, W. A. (1983). A review of the Screening Test for Developmental Apraxia of Speech. *Language, Speech, and Services in Schools, 14,* 202–209.

Hardy, J. C. (1983). *Cerebral palsy.* Englewood Cliffs, NJ: Prentice-Hall.

Haynes, S. (1985). Developmental apraxia: Symptoms and treatment. In D. F. Johns (Ed.), *Clinical management of neurogenic communication disorders* (2nd ed.) (pp. 259–266). Boston: Little, Brown.

Hiskey, M. S. (1966). *Hiskey-Nebraska Test of Learning Aptitude.* Lincoln, NE: Union College Press.

Hixon, T., & Hardy, J. (1964). Restricted motility of the speech articulators in cerebral palsy. *Journal of Speech and Hearing Disorders, 29,* 293–306.

Ingram, T. T. S. (1962). Clinical significance of the infantile feeding reflexes. *Developmental Medicine and Child Neurology, 4,* 159–169.

Jaffe, M. B. (1986). Neurological impairment of speech production: Assessment and treatment. In J. M. Costello & A. L. Holland (Eds.), *Handbook of speech and language disorders* (pp. 157–186). San Diego: College Hill Press.

Kent, R., & Netsell, R. (1975). A case study of an ataxic dysarthric: Cineradiographic and spectographic. *Journal of Speech and Hearing Disorders, 40,* 115–134.

Kent, R., & Netsell, R. (1978). Articulatory abnormalities in athetoid cerebral palsy. *Journal of Speech and Hearing Disorders, 43,* 353–373.

Kramer, S. (1989). Radiologic examination of the swallowing impaired child. *Dysphagia, 3,* 117–125.

Lenn, N. J., & Freinkel, A. (1989). Facial sparing in patients with prenatal onset hemiparesis. *Pediatric Neurology, 5,* 291–295.

Lotz, W. K., & Netsell, R. (1989). Velopharyngeal management for a child with dysarthria and cerebral palsy. In K. M. Yorkston & D. R. Beukelman (Eds.), *Recent advances in clinical dysarthria* (pp. 139–143). Boston: Little, Brown.

Love, R. J., & Fitzgerald, M. (1984). Is the diagnosis of developmental apraxia of speech valid? *Australian Journal of Human Communication Disorders, 12,* 170–178.

Love, R. J., Hagerman, E. L., & Tiami E. G. (1980). Speech performance, dysphagia and oral reflexes in cerebral palsy. *Journal of Speech and Hearing Disorders, 45,* 59–75.

Love, R. J., & Webb, W. G. (1996). *Neurology for the speech-language pathologist* (3rd ed.). Boston: Butterworth.

McDonald, E. T. (1968). *Screening Deep Test of Articulation.* Pittsburgh: Stanwick House.

McDonald, E. T., & Chance, B., Jr. (1964). *Cerebral palsy.* Englewood Cliffs, NJ: Prentice-Hall.

Meyer, L. A. (1983). *A study of vocal, prosodic and articulatory parameters of the speech of spastic and athetotic cerebral palsied individuals.* Unpublished doctoral dissertation, Vanderbilt University, Nashville, TN.

Morris, S. E. (1982). *Prespeech Assessment Scale: A rating scale for the measurement of pre-speech behaviors from birth through two years.* Clifton, NJ: Preston.

Morris, S. E., & Klien, M. D. (1987). *Pre-feeding skills.* Tucson, AZ: Therapy Skill Builders.

Mysak, E. D. (1980). *Neurospeech therapy for the cerebral palsied.* New York: Teachers College Press.

Mysak, E. D. (1987). Assessment of speech readiness in cerebral palsy. *Seminars in Speech and Language, 8,* 43–56.

Neilson, P. D., Andrews, G., Guitar, B. E., Quinn, P. T. (1979). Tonic stretch reflexes in lip, tongue and jaw muscles. *Brain Research, 178,* 311–327.

Neilson, P. D., & O'Dwyer, N. J. (1981). Physiopathology of dysarthria in cerebral palsy. *Journal of Neurology, Neurosurgery and Psychiatry, 44,* 1013–1019.

Netsell, R. (1969). Evaluation of velopharyngeal function in dysarthria. *Journal of Speech and Hearing Disorders, 34,* 113–122.

Netsell, R., Lotz, W. K., & Barlow, S. (1989). A speech physiology examination for individuals with dysarthria. In K. M. Yorkston & D. R. Beukelman (Eds.), *Recent advances in clinical dysarthria* (pp. 3–37). Boston: Little, Brown.

Palmer, N. (1947). Studies in clinical techniques: II. Normalization of chewing, sucking and swallowing reflexes in cerebral palsy: A home program. *Journal of Speech Disorders, 12,* 415–418.

Platt, J. F., Andrews, G., Young, M., & Quinn, P. T. (1980). Dysarthria in cerebral palsy: I. Intelligibility and articulatory impairment. *Journal of Speech and Hearing Research, 23,* 28–38.

Robbins, J., & Klee, T. (1987). Clinical assessment of oropharyngeal motor development in young children. *Journal of Speech and Hearing Disorders, 52,* 271–277.

Shane, H. C., & Bashir, A. S. (1980). Election criteria for adoption of an augmentative communication system: Preliminary considerations. *Journal of Speech and Hearing Disorders, 45,* 408–414.

Sheppard, J. J. (1964). Craniopharyngeal motor patterns in dysarthria associated with cerebral palsy. *Journal of Speech and Hearing Research, 7,* 373–380.

Sheppard, J. J. (1987). Assessment of oral motor behaviors in cerebral palsy. *Seminars in Speech and Language, 8,* 57–70.

Stark, R. E. (1985). Dysarthria in children. In J. B. Darby (Ed.), *Speech and language evaluation in neurology: Childhood disorders* (pp. 185–217). New York: Grune & Stratton.

Thompson, C. K. (1988). Articulation disorders in the child with neurogenic pathology. In N. J. Lass, L. V. McReynolds, J. L. Northern, & D. E. Yoder (Eds.), *Handbook of speech-language pathology and audiology* (pp. 548–591). Toronto: B. C. Decker.

Tuchman, D. N. (1989). Cough, choke sputter: The evaluation of the child with dysfunctional swallowing. *Dysphagia, 3,* 111–116.

Vitali, G. J. (1986). *Test of Oral Structures and Functions.* East Aurora, NY: Slosson Education Publications.

Wechsler, D. (1974). *Manual for the Wechsler Intelligence Scale for Children—Revised.* New York: Psychological Corp.

Westlake, H. (1951). Muscle training for cerebral palsied speech cases. *Journal of Speech and Hearing Disorders, 16,* 103–109.

Westlake, H., & Rutherford, D. (1961). *Speech therapy for the cerebral palsied.* Chicago: National Easter Seal Society for Crippled Children and Adults.

Wilson, B. D., & Davidovicz, H. M. (1987). Neuropsychological assessment of the child with cerebral palsy. *Seminars in Speech and Language, 8,* 1–18.

Workinger, M. S. (1988). Feeding disorders in the infant and young child. In D. Yoder & R. Kent (Eds.), *Decision making in speech-language pathology* (pp. 110–111). Toronto: B. C. Decker.

Yorkston, K. M., & Beukelman, D. R. (1980). A clinician judged technique for quantifying dysarthric speech based on single word intelligibility. *Journal of Communication Disorders, 13,* 15–31.

Yorkston, K. M., & Beukelman, D. R. (1981). *Assessment of intelligibility of dysarthric speech.* Tigard, OR: C C Publications.

7

Issues in Speech Management of Childhood Dysarthria

*Once goals are defined a comprehensive management
program must be devised choosing from several available
approaches. No "right" answers exist . . .*
—JANET LORD, 1984

Introduction

Prespeech Oral-Motor Training and Early Intervention
 Oral Motor Training in Infant Feeding • Early Intervention

Later Oral-Motor Management
 Oral-Motor Exercises • Drooling Therapy

Technology in Childhood Dysarthria
 *Biofeedback Technology • Communication Aid Technology •
 New Developments*

INTRODUCTION

Speech-language pathology students and working clinicians are often confused when faced with the current state of affairs concerning approaches to
speech management in childhood dysarthria. The field is dominated by con-

141

flicting approaches to treatment and strongly held opinions, often unsupported by empirical data, as to the "right" approach to management of the child with a neurologic speech impairment. The purpose of this chapter is to point out the several issues surrounding current management approaches and to suggest which of these approaches seem the most logical and appropriate at the present time. Six topics will be discussed: (1) oral-motor training in infant feeding, (2) early intervention efficacy, (3) oral-motor exercises, (4) drooling therapy, (5) biofeedback technology, and (6) communication aid technology.

PRESPEECH ORAL-MOTOR TRAINING AND EARLY INTERVENTION

Oral-Motor Training in Infant Feeding

One of the most critical issues in speech management is whether feeding programs should be a major focus of oral-motor training for infants and young children with suspected or verified cerebral damage. As indicated in the previous chapter, pioneer experts in child dysarthria often advocated programs in oral-motor training in which feeding was a means of improving oral-motor function for speech. More recently the profession has rejected the concept of a direct correlation between oral movements in speech and eating behavior (Jaffe, 1986). This rejection was fostered by the early pivotal study by Hixon and Hardy (1964), who found differences between speech and non-speech diadochokinetic movement in dysarthric children and argued that speech movement control was mediated at a different level in the nervous system than was nonspeech movement control. Although the statistical analysis that allowed this conclusion to be drawn has been questioned (Abbs & Rosenbek, 1986), it is clear that the infantile reflexes involved in chewing and swallowing behavior are mediated at brain-stem levels, not at the cortical level of oral-motor control as is speech (Dubner, Sessle, & Storey, 1978). It is likely, as Hardy (1983) points out, that improvement of infantile chewing and swallowing behavior in no way contributes to the development of neural networks for speech production. The work of Love, Hagerman, & Tiami (1980) supports the view that oral reflexes and chewing and swallowing behavior are relatively independent of speech production mechanisms. They found no strong and systematic relationship between either the severity of persisting abnormal oral reflexes and speech performance or the number of dysphagic symptoms. Dysphagic symptoms were slightly better predictors of the severity of dysarthria than was the presence of persisting oral reflexes in the 60 cerebral-palsied subjects studied, but neither was strongly correlated with the severity of dysarthria. In brief, the available research to date makes the issue of prespeech oral-motor training a controversial one.

Although the evidence from recent studies of the development of mandibular action in normal children suggests that motor coordination for speech activities is clearly different than it is for nonspeech activities (Moore & Ruark, 1996), it does not completely contradict the need for prespeech muscle training of lips, tongue, jaw, and soft palate in such motor activities as chewing, swallowing, sucking, blowing, and oral muscle diadochokinesis in orally involved cerebral palsied children. It is clear that the muscles for speech are also involved in nonspeech behavior.

Early Intervention

In recent years there has been a consistent trend toward early programmatic intervention with the infant with verified or suspected cerebral injury. Most early intervention programs have been designed on principles of physical therapy management derived from a Bobath neurodevelopmental therapy approach (Bobath, 1967, 1971, 1980; Bobath & Bobath, 1972). Infants are typically enrolled in these programs within the first year of life, often as early as two months of age (Erenberg, 1984).

Many, but not all, of the speech-language pathologists who advocate oral-motor training through feeding are also proponents of neurodevelopmental therapy (NDT) and view feeding management as part of a total neurodevelopmental program (Alexander, 1987a & b; Morris, 1987). Morris (1987), for instance, emphasizes a comprehensive program encompassing a variety of developmental activities. These include facilitating normal developmental motor sequences as soon as possible. An intensive study of body postures, motor reactions, and oral-motor behavior is conducted. Bobath (1971, 1980) devised methods for modifying abnormal reflex postures and motor reactions; these methods of therapy are implemented as early as is feasible. Parents are involved intensively in the management of their child. They are instructed in the use of normalizing postures and appropriate handling methods for their child. Morris (1987) indicates that several postures for handling children are dependent upon the specific situation, and each of these must be carefully determined. In addition, emphasis is also placed on auditory, visual, tactile, and other sensory stimulation to increase the sensorimotor awareness of the child. Oral-motor training specifically involves reduction of abnormal oral reactions, such as abnormal reflexes, and the facilitation of normal prespeech and feeding behaviors in the child.

Training in Prespeech and Feeding Management.   Many university training programs have been reluctant to incorporate instruction on feeding management into their curricula because of the controversial nature of the relationship between feeding behavior and speech development as well as the lack of published documentation of the effectiveness of neurodevelopmental speech programs. Such programs, because of their comprehensive approach to management in terms of physical therapy, are highly specialized and demand intensive special training. Many of the skills required, such as identification and management of abnormal primitive and postural reflexes, are not in the repertoire of most speech-language pathologists. University programs are hesitant to provide such highly specialized training for disorders of low incidence.

However, it is abundantly clear that dysphagia, and to a lesser degree abnormal oral reflexes, are common and significant disorders in neurologically impaired children (Love et al., 1980; Sheppard, 1964). Appropriate early management of dysphagia and abnormal oral reflexes has several advantages for the child at risk. Nutritional intake will be improved at a critical period in infancy, difficult and prolonged feeding sessions will be made easier for both child and caregiver, and in all likelihood the control of oral movements will be made more normal. This improved oral-motor control then can be utilized for improved speech production when speech has its onset.

Neurodevelopmental therapists currently are providing leadership in prespeech feeding management, and in many instances, it is apparent that the neurodevelopmental approach, as a whole, is becoming the therapy of choice worldwide for treating neurologically impaired and at-risk infants.

As a result, speech-language pathologists often find themselves playing significant roles in these programs. The therapeutic feeding program is usually carried out by one of two professionals in these settings—the speech-language pathologist or the occupational therapist. It is certainly desirable for the speech-language pathologist to play a major role in this program since he or she has had the added special training in areas of communication skills for infants and young children. For the speech-language pathologist who has not been provided with prespeech and feeding coursework in his or her university training program, there are several available postgraduate workshops presented by NDT experts. In addition, there is a substantial body of literature available to speech-language pathologists who need assistance in providing techniques of prespeech oral-motor training and feeding therapy. In the Suggested Reading section at the end of this chapter, a list of articles, chapters, and therapy manuals dealing with techniques in feeding therapy are given. Space does not allow a review of the extensive literature now available in this area, but special mention should be made of the excellent manual *Prefeeding Skills* (Morris & Klien, 1987). It is a comprehensive, practical, well-illustrated guide for speech pathologists and parents alike who are interested in developing a therapeutic feeding program for the neurologically impaired infant.

As feeding programs make a resurgence in the plan for speech management of the neurologically impaired child (Alexander, 1987a & b; Morris, 1982, 1985, 1987; Morris & Klien, 1987), it is important to point out that feeding therapy may achieve only limited success in attaining the ultimate goal of more normal speech unless serious attention is paid to the identification and facilitation of prespeech sound-making during the period of oral-motor training in feeding (Stark, 1985). Emphasis must be placed specifically on the child's early sound-making attempts. Early sound-making must be imitated, reinforced, and stimulated frequently by the caregiver. Certainly until data is available to the contrary, it appears logical that the optimal program should give equal weight to feeding therapy and stimulation of developmental sequences of early vocal utterances. The parallel programs of oral-motor training in feeding therapy and stimulation of developmental sound-making are consistent with a neurology of dual circuit for feeding behavior and speech performance (Hardy, 1983).

Early Intervention Efficacy. Since specific data is as yet unavailable concerning the value of prespeech and feeding programs in infants, one may ask how effective neurodevelopmental early intervention is in general in resolving early neurologic symptoms. Despite growing international acceptance of these programs, there is limited published evidence of their efficacy. Over the past quarter of a century there have been repeated questions raised by the medical community about the merits of these programs and the lack of scientific evidence supporting them (Bax & MacKeith, 1967; Browne, 1966; Ferry, 1981; Pearson, 1982; Taft, 1972).

The rationale for these programs is derived in part from an early statement of Bobath (1967). She believes that early intervention with at-risk children is based on the following principles:

1. The nervous system of the infant displays more plasticity than that of an older child.
2. Early treatment provides critical sensorimotor experiences that decrease the learning and reinforcement of abnormal motor patterns.
3. Early treatment capitalizes on the fact that abnormal postural patterns resulting from cerebral injury often are less severe than later ones and can be remediated more quickly.
4. Contractures (permanent muscle contraction) may be prevented by early treatment.

Early studies of the ability of neurodevelopmental therapy for infants to reduce or reverse the symptoms of neurologic impairment were plagued by contradictory and inconclusive results, often because of lack of random control groups (Kong, 1966; Scherzer, Mike, & Ilson, 1976; Wright & Nicholson, 1973). The most recent study (Katona, 1989) suggests moderate success in training cerebral-palsied infants to activate and maintain synchronous movements in all extremities. Forty-five percent of the infants in the program who were motor retarded during the first 16 to 24 months of life reached completely normal motor development with rehabilitation. Another 22% needed further motor rehabilitation during the second year of life. Their motor retardation lasted up to three or four years of age and longer in some children. In 75% of this subsample, motor retardation was resolved. In the remaining 25%, motor symptoms remained and hampered sitting, walking, and motor flexibility. The remainder of the total sample, 32%, did not reach a necessary level of motor ability to move about without support. These children ultimately became motor retarded. Katona readily admits that a definitive test of the efficacy of his infant neurorehabilitation program must await a randomized control series. Therefore, the results, flawed by lack of randomized controls, must be viewed with caution; but they suggest that early intervention probably plays an important role in motor rehabilitation of impaired infants.

In addition, it has been pointed out (Russman & Romnes, 1998) that in reviewing the beneficial effects of any physical therapy program, more than motor outcome must be considered. The psychological impact of rearing a disabled child can be devastating. Frequently, the specific diagnosis does not cause as much stress to a parent as does the dependency of the child on the parent to help him or her accomplish the activities of daily living. In such cases, a therapeutic program may be extremely helpful, not necessarily in stimulating development but rather in offering parents easier ways to work with their child. Faced with the present inconclusive evidence about the efficacy of early infant neurorehabilitation, speech-language pathologists and other professionals are probably wise to follow the advice of Browne (1966, p. 473) about recommendations for early intervention: "When the outcome of doing nothing is uncertain, all cases should be treated without exception. Most . . . correct themselves spontaneously, but if they are left to see which will and which won't, there is a residue of disasters."

LATER ORAL-MOTOR MANAGEMENT

Oral-Motor Exercises

The use of muscle training programs to improve the efficiency of the oral mechanism has become a controversial topic in the management of dysarthric speakers (Yorkston, Beukelman, & Bell, 1986). In past decades, muscle training programs were widely advocated by speech-language pathologists in treatment programs for the childhood dysarthrias of cerebral palsy (Cass, 1951; McDonald & Chance, 1964; Westlake & Rutherford, 1961).

Muscle training has long been accepted as a critical modality of treatment in physical medicine and rehabilitation, but few clinical research studies have focused on its effect in childhood dysarthria. Krusen, Kottke, and Ellwood (1982) indicate that general muscle training programs can increase muscle strength, mass, endurance, and length. Muscle training improves sensory feedback and control. It develops coordinated patterns to accomplish tasks and, under certain circumstances, helps nerves regain lost capacities. Muscles, however, must be exercised in specific ways to achieve each of these goals. To increase strength and mass, a muscle must contract to nearly its maximum potential while working against resistance for relatively few repetitions. Muscles exercised repeatedly against low resistance with numerous contractions will improve endurance. Increasing muscle length or contractibility involves stretching the muscle. Coordinated muscle patterns must be learned and practiced repeatedly before they can be incorporated into a complex motor pattern. Generally, attempts to increase or modify sensory function of muscles rely on procedures that involve tactile or electrical stimulation.

Conflicting Research Findings.   Muscle training programs to improve nonspeech oral muscle function in the cerebral-palsied were recommended by several speech-language pathologists in the past. For example, Westlake and Rutherford (1961) advocated increasing nonspeech motion rates to improve speaking rate and used diadochokinetic muscle drills to increase the range of motion of oral muscles. Described and illustrated in their publication were techniques that provided resistance to oral movement in an attempt to strengthen muscles. Hixon and Hardy (1964) of course denied that training in nonspeech activities had a major effect on motor control for speech; but in a more recent study with spastic individuals, Barlow and Abbs (1986) found that movement and force control of oral facial muscles were highly related to speech intelligibility. In contrast, from their research with cerebral-palsied speakers, O'Dwyer, Neilson, Guitar, Quinn, and Andrews (1983) doubt that muscle weakness or pathological muscle imbalance of oral or mandibular muscles is critical to speech movements.

The conflicting research findings concerning muscle weakness and other types of oral-motor performance and their effects on speech suggest that careful analysis of muscle strength and movement rates in a given dysarthric child is probably the only reasonable guide for recommending oral exercises to increase muscle strength or movements. Even if muscle weakness is apparent, one must attempt to determine whether this weakness interferes with speech function (Yorkston et al., 1986). Barlow and Abbs (1983) have shown that only 10 to 20% of the maximum force of lip movements is needed for speech. Movement rates, precision, and coordination of movement are apparently more critical to speech performance than is muscle strength.

Children with flaccid dysarthria, of course, may benefit from direct strengthening exercises using resistance. Children with spasticity also show muscle weakness (Barlow & Abbs, 1986) and respond to strengthening exercises. Dyskinetic and ataxic dysarthric children are less likely to show significant muscle weakness. However, oral-motor exercises that increase articulator movement rates or exercises that increase precision of movement may be of more importance to child dysarthrics than are muscle strengthening drills.

Care must be taken to plan exercise regimes that are not judged as excessively monotonous or frustrating. Cerebral-palsied children have often viewed speech therapy sessions as negative experiences because of an overemphasis on oral motor drills (Richardson, 1972).

In summary, current management programs for childhood dysarthria are likely to use a broad spectrum of techniques for improving speech. Oral exercises generally are given limited prominence in current dysarthric management programs as compared to their prominence in past programs (Yorkston et al., 1986).

Drooling Therapy

Excessive drooling is often a chronic and difficult problem associated with childhood dysarthria. The speech-language pathologist often is required to assume the treatment of the problem or is expected to make a recommendation for its management by other experts. The management of drooling also remains controversial because no obvious treatment of choice has emerged from years of treating neurologically impaired children.

Drooling is inconvenient, embarrassing, and socially stigmatizing to the child. Chronic drooling commonly requires that children wear infant bibs or frequently change damp clothing. It interferes with the use of books, toys, and other items in school, home, or therapy and often makes it difficult to use alternate or augmentative communication devices. The public sometimes associates drooling with signs of mental retardation, so the child who drools chronically is often thought to be retarded even if he is actually free of cognitive limitations. Furthermore, drooling children no doubt receive less affection and physical contact because of their dampness and the occasional foul smell associated with drooling.

Chronic drooling has usually been thought to be associated primarily with poor motor control of the pharyngeal stage of swallowing. Other factors, however, may play a significant role in its persistence in a child. Characteristics such as poor lip control, open bite, missing teeth, facial weakness, sensory loss of the lower face, and abundant secretion brought about by saliva-producing foods all contribute to the problem. Despite the fact that the relevant contributing factors are often recognized, it remains difficult to significantly decrease or completely eliminate salivary incontinence.

Management for the problem has, for the most part, been behavioral. Drooling masks, behavior modification techniques to condition swallowing, and ostentatious bibs have been used to protect the child's clothing or to shame him or her into an awareness and control of the salivary incontinence. Medical and surgical approaches generally have been viewed as radical, but several of these techniques have been employed with varying success. These include tympanic neurectomy, radiation of the salivary glands, and direct surgical intervention. A plastic surgeon, Theodore Wilkie (1967), described an approach in which the parotid glands were repositioned so that the flow of saliva was redirected. The procedure was not always completely successful (Wilkie & Brody, 1977). Brown and his colleagues (1985) modified the Wilkie procedure and reported the results of a selected sample of 10 children 6 to 11 years of age. The amount of drool was carefully measured pre- and post-operatively. Following surgery, drooling was reported to be substantially reduced in all children in the sample. It was reported that all children benefited psychologically in that they received positive comments on their appearance and received more physical affection. Other drooling children wished to undergo surgery when they saw the results. Positive results have not been reported as yet in terms of improved feeding or articulation. It is speculated by Brown and his colleagues that drier contact points for articulators will provide more sensory information for articulation. This surgical approach appears promising; however, it must be documented more fully before it becomes the treatment of choice for this unresolved problem. It appears that a problem as extreme as constant drooling may demand a cure as radical as surgery.

Of all the therapy techniques suggested in the first edition of this book, surgery for severe drooling drew the most criticism. Several physicians argued that parotid gland repositioning interfered with the normal cleansing process that saliva performed. However, an experienced dental consultant suggested that in a severe drooler with cerebral palsy, good oral hygiene techniques, including adequate brushing and regular fluoride treatment, rarely occurred in the home. With such a dental program in place, he noted, it was highly likely that radical surgery for control of drooling would be successful (R. Swang, D.D.S., Personal communication, August 1998.)

TECHNOLOGY IN CHILDHOOD DYSARTHRIA

Biofeedback Technology

Biofeedback techniques are clearly useful habilitation techniques in neurologic impairment. These techniques have been reported to be used more widely with adult dysarthrics than with child dysarthrics. Netsell and Daniel (1979), for instance, report that adults improve their control of individual aspects of speech production when given biofeedback. They assert that biofeedback allows the individual to focus on specific aspects of a more general problem by providing simplified and instantaneous comparisons between disordered muscle action and normal muscle action, Medical experts, however, still consider biofeedback experimental in use with neurologically impaired children (Lord, 1984).

Deficient motor control in cerebral palsy, however, may be secondary to inadequate proprioceptive sensory function or to inadequate inhibition of muscle contraction. Spastic muscles create resistance to voluntary contraction of agonists by simultaneous contraction of the antagonist muscle. Biofeedback provides visual or auditory signals to convey proprioceptive information or knowledge of the degree of muscle relaxation, and there is evidence that head control, individual muscle spasm, and specific articulation movements may be controlled by biofeedback (Neilson & McCaughey, 1982; Netsell & Daniel, 1979; Woolridge & Russell, 1976).

The biofeedback technique is extremely promising and deserves more research attention in childhood motor speech problems. Motivation and intelligence appear to play a role in its success in that there may be limitations due to poor motivation and lowered intelligence in some neurologically impaired children (Lord, 1984). Usually, biofeedback techniques have been employed in combination with other techniques to create a total speech management program for dysarthria (Yorkston et al., 1986).

Communication Aid Technology

Some children with motor speech disabilities present a severe motor impairment with a poor prognosis for developing oral speech. For the dysarthric child who is speechless or severely unintelligible, augmentative or alternate communication devices have long been a viable option to oral speech. As early as the 1950s in U.S. hospital-schools for the cerebral-palsied, simple picture boards, word boards, or a combination of the two were tried with the anarthric child who could use extremity pointers or head pointers to indicate words and pictures for communication purposes. Materials and articles describing communication board options began to appear in the literature in the next two decades (Dixon & Curry, 1965; Feallock, 1958; Goldberg & Fenton, n.d.; McDonald & Schutz, 1973; Vicker, 1974). Descriptions of other types of communication systems, including simple electronic devices and sign language procedures, also appeared at this time with recommendations for use with anarthric, dyspraxic, and mentally retarded children. These publications provided the field of communication disorders with evidence that even simple augmentative communication devices had distinct advantages for many neurologically impaired children. Supplemental and assistive communication systems increase attention, reduce frustration, and raise motivational levels. Shane (1987) points out that increased experience with these alternate and supplemental modes of communication has clarified their many advantages. They may serve as an expressive language system that is a substitute for spoken language, or they may enhance existing expressive speech. They often improve language comprehension and serve as an organizer of language, which reduces notable discrepancies between comprehension and expression in language.

Historically, after communication boards were in wide use, simple automated communication devices became available. These allowed literate children with motor speech disabilities to communicate using electric typewriters or simple scanning devices. Pointers of various types allowed the motor-impaired child to write independently or prepare messages in advance. Scanning devices allowed those with extreme disability to make their needs known or to express their ideas.

Scanning devices generally are composed of a display surface, an indicator, and an operating switch. Information is exposed on the display surface in an organized fashion that allows the child to conveniently access intended information. An indicator, usually in the form of an arrow, light, or cursor, is powered by electronic switches. Detailed descriptions of scanning devices and other communication technology can be found in Musselwhite and St. Louis (1988).

Other types of communication aids based on more sophisticated technology have become widely available in the past decade. These are categorized as microprocessors for individual use. These high-technology systems provide synthetic or digitized voice output with rate enhancement. These communication aids are usually called **dedicated systems** because they are for the personal use of only a single disabled person.

The widespread use of the personal computer with customized software and hardware has presented another option for the communicatively disabled that is in wide use today. Present-day computer technology has been able to reduce some of the delay problems present in many currently used augmentative communication systems. Dedicated software programs are available that allow letter and linguistic form prediction, thus speeding the rate of message transmission. Software programs that allow accessing of specialized vocabulary, which speeds the rate of message transmission, also are available. Systems that provide spoken output can bypass the need for specialized symbol systems like *Blissymbolics* (Kates & McNaughton, 1974), which is in use internationally with cerebral-palsied children.

Both digitized and synthesized speech can be created by the present-day computer. Vocabulary represented in digitized speech, however, must be developed in advance. It does not allow phonemes to be combined into words, so the vocabulary is fixed or permanent. On the other hand, synthesized speech systems allow infinite creation of messages with a finite set of symbols. The quality of speech on most available units does not yet produce a voice that is age and gender appropriate (Shane, 1987). Thus, a degree of social stigma probably will be associated with the use of such a device, but the advantages to communication may outweigh the negative reactions surrounding the system.

The computer clearly provides substantial potential for severely motor speech disabled children. It can produce reasonably rapid nonvocal communication and can also provide voice output in some instances. For the speechless individual, the computer usually becomes more than a communication aid. In certain circumstances it enhances the learning processes, and in other instances it ultimately serves as the basis of a vocation for the severely handicapped adult.

Not all speech experts have viewed computers or other assistive communication devices as a panacea for the motor speech disabled. Hardy (1983), Netsell, Lotz, and Barlow (1989), Thompson (1988), and Yorkston et al. (1986) advocate using augmentative communication at necessary points in the overall speech management plan for the dysarthric person, but when at all possible, they propose aiming for oral speech as a primary goal with limited assistance from communication aids unless the child is definitely destined to be a nonoral communicator.

Thompson (1988) points out that few speech-language pathologists have actually presented data to document the benefits of providing nonspeech communication systems to nonspeaking and dysarthric children. Culp (1987) has suggested that communication boards are often rejected, and Udwin (1987) reports that in Britain, where *Blissymbolics* and sign language are widely used with cerebral-palsied children, most programs use these systems merely in artificial teaching situations. Formal usage of the systems is only a few minutes per week, and the children generally do not use these nonvocal systems widely in communicative situations where they might be useful. Real-life applications are not being taught, it appears.

The decision to recommend communication technology for a child with motor speech disability is a critical one and careful consideration must be given to the decision process leading to the election of an augmentative or alternate communication system. Many authors have considered the decision process; the work of Shane and Bashir (1980) is particularly helpful in that they have formalized the decision process into a branching decision matrix. This decision matrix is presented in a modified form in Figure 7-1.

The Shane-Bashir decision matrix is to be considered a clinical aid, since the final decision for electing augmentative communication must be a blend of clinical art and science. The decision matrix consists of 10 categories or levels (Levels I–X), the specific components of each category, and branching alternatives. The final decision is expressed in three options: (1) elect, (2) delay, or (3) reject the concept of an augmentative or alternate communication system.

Generally, the Shane-Bashir decision matrix is a well-conceived clinical aid providing the speech-language pathologist with a format to help in the decision-making process. However, one category in the original matrix is of concern. In the original matrix, Level II Oral Reflex Factors indicated that the obligatory persistence of oral reflexes in the child can, in isolation, lead to an immediate decision to elect an augmentative or alternate communication system. Shane and Bashir believe that no other factor has such a powerful influence on the election of communication technology because many authorities in the field of childhood dysarthria believe that persisting oral reflexes suggest a very poor prognosis for oral speech development. In the presence of abnormal oral reflexes, then, the original matrix suggested that augmentative communication be elected at Level II and other levels be ignored, with the exception of Level X, which features a discussion of the implementation of augmentative or alternate communication. Research by Love et al. (1980), however, has suggested that the presence of persisting oral reflexes does not necessarily predict a poor prognosis for the development of oral speech in cerebral-palsied individuals. The speech of these individuals was dysarthric in most cases, but the persisting oral reflexes did not always seem to contribute to the level of severity of the dysarthria. In fact, the presence of dysphagic symptoms was a much better predictor of severity of dysarthria. Hence, Figure 7-1 has been adapted to indicate that the presence of abnormal oral reflexes may be an uncertain factor in the election of augmentative or alternate communication and that other factors considered in the decision matrix should be given considerable weight in the final decision to elect communication technology.

In brief, despite the growing interest and greater application of communication aid technology in the area of childhood motor speech disability, many of its potential uses and benefits remain controversial because of limited researching of outcomes. In the hands of knowledgeable and thoughtful clinicians (Buzolich, 1987; Montgomery, 1987), the use of these devices appears particularly beneficial—especially where usable and acceptable oral speech has not developed naturally. For the selected child, communication aids are very effective and appropriate. In most dysarthric children, some type of oral speech will remain the goal.

LEVEL I   COGNITIVE FACTORS

At least Stage V sensorimotor intelligence?

At least 18 months mental age, or ability to recognize at least at photograph level?

YES   →   Go to II

NO   →   Delay

LEVEL II   ORAL REFLEX FACTORS

Persistent (1) Rooting, (2) Gag, (3) Bite, (4) Suckle/Swallow, or (5) Jaw
Extension Reflex?

UNCERTAIN   →   Go to III

NO   →   Continue to III

LEVEL III   LANGUAGE AND MOTOR SPEECH PRODUCTION FACTORS

A Is there a discrepancy between receptive and expressive skills?

YES   →   Go to III B

NO   →   Go to V

B Is the discrepancy explained predominantly on the basis of a motor speech
disorder?

YES   →   Go to V

NO   →   Go to III C

UNCERTAIN   →   Go to IV

C Is the discrepancy explained predominantly on the basis of an expressive
language disorder?

YES   →   Go to VII

NO   →   Go to VI

UNCERTAIN   →   Go to V

LEVEL IV   MOTOR SPEECH—SOME CONTRIBUTING FACTORS

Presence of neuromuscular involvement affecting postural tone and/or postural
stability?

Presence of praxic disturbance?

Vocal production consists primarily of vowel production?

Vocal production consists primarily of undifferentiated sounds?

History of eating problems?

Excessive drooling?

YES   →   Evidence to support motor speech involvement (Go to V)

NO   →   Evidence against motor speech involvement (Go to V)

LEVEL V   PRODUCTION—SOME CONTRIBUTING FACTORS

Speech unintelligible except to family and immediate friends?

Predominant mode of communication is through pointing, gesture, facial-body
affect?

Predominance of single-word utterances?

Frustration associated with inability to speak?

YES   →   (Evidence to ELECT) Go to VII

NO   →   (Evidence to DELAY OR REJECT)
Go to VII

FIGURE 7-1   Decision Matrix for Election of Communication Technology

Adapted from "Election criteria for the adoption of an augmentative communication system: Preliminary considerations" by H. C. Shane and A. S. Bashir (1980), *Journal of Speech and Hearing Disorders, 45,* 409.

LEVEL VI EMOTIONAL FACTORS

A History of precipitous loss of expressive speech?
   YES → Go to VIII
   NO   → Go to VI B

B Speaks to selected persons or refuses to speak?
   YES → Go to VIII
   NO   → Go to V

LEVEL VII CHRONOLOGICAL AGE FACTORS

A Chronological age less than 3 years?
   YES → Go to VIII A

B Chronological age between 3 and 5 years?
   YES → Go to VIII A

C Chronological age greater than 5 years?
   YES → Go to VIII A

LEVEL VIII PREVIOUS THERAPY FACTORS

A Has had previous therapy?
   YES → Go to VIII B
   NO   → Go to IX, weigh evidence—(DELAY with trial therapy or
            ELECT) Go to X

B Previous therapy appropriate?
   YES → Go to VIII C
   NO   → DELAY with trial therapy

C Therapy progress too slow to enable effective communication?
   YES → ELECT → Go to X
   NO   → DELAY → Continue therapy

D Therapy appropriately withheld?
   YES → ELECT → Go to X
   NO   → DELAY with trial therapy

LEVEL IX PREVIOUS THERAPY—SOME CONTRIBUTING FACTORS

Able to imitate (with accuracy) speech sounds or words, gross motor or oral
motor movements?
   YES → (Evidence to DELAY) Go to VIII
   NO   → (Evidence to ELECT) Go to VIII

LEVEL X IMPLEMENTATION FACTORS—ENVIRONMENT

Family willing to implement (use, allow to be introduced) Augmentative
Communication System recommendation?
   YES → IMPLEMENT
   NO   → COUNSEL

New Developments

Since the first edition of this text, there have been several reports on the treatment efficacy of augmentative communication technology for cerebral-palsied individuals (Yorkston, 1996). Many systems for augmentative and alternate communication have been developed and compared. Angelo (1996) studied three scanning modes used by cerebral-palsied persons and found that the effectiveness of each mode depended on the type of cerebral palsy. According to Light and Lindsay (1992), some methods of message encoding increase learning while others do not. Clearly, letter encoding is superior to iconic encoding. Further, McNaughton and Tawney (1993) have shown that two spelling techniques have approximately the same learning rates but one is retained better.

Training in the use of alternate and augmentative systems with cerebral-palsied individuals using partners has recently been explored. Light, Datillo, English, Guiterrez, and Hartz (1992) found that turn-taking and initiation patterns were more reciprocal between the individuals and their partners after training. However, Bedrosian, Hoag, Johnson, and Calculator (1998) studied the effects of aided message length and partner feedback on communicative competence in cerebral-palsied individuals and found ratings of communicative competence were not affected by aided message length nor did partner feedback have an effect on ratings of communicative competence. Light, Binger, Agate, and Ramsay (1999) found that teaching partner-focused questions to cerebral-palsied and other individuals who use augmentative and alternate communication was generally successful. All the participants in the instruction program reported high levels of satisfaction with the program, and members of the general public judged the majority of the participants to be more competent communicators after instruction.

In summary, the growing interest in carefully researching the several variables that effect success in use of augmentative and alternate communication techniques in persons with severe communication problems is noteworthy. Certainly much more research is needed to fine-tune computer use with the severely impaired individual with cerebral palsy.

SUMMARY

This chapter discusses six topics in the management of the child who has dysarthria or is at risk for the condition: (1) oral-motor training in infant feeding, (2) early intervention efficacy, (3) oral-motor exercises, (4) drooling therapy, (5) biofeedback technology, and (6) communication aid technology. To a greater or lesser degree, each of these topics is controversial or at least engenders varied opinions from the professionals managing the neurologically impaired child with a speech disorder. The discussions illustrate the point that speech-language pathologists do not yet have all the "right" answers concerning therapy for the child with dysarthria. These topics are significant because the child with dysarthria often presents one of the most serious speech problems in the field of communication disorders, and management programs for the child must be of proven effectiveness. The controversy surrounding these topics must be resolved by research before the treatment of childhood dysarthria can be considered totally effective and scientifically based.

Recent approaches to the area of management of childhood dysarthria suggest that current management of childhood motor speech disability probably is more successful than it has been in the past because of the use of early intervention programs and recent technology. Special attention has been given to the rather intensive study of the computer technology that has been used with the severely communicatively disabled cerebral-palsied individual since the last edition of this book.

SUGGESTED READING

Thompson, C. K. (1988). Articulation disorders in the child with neurogenic pathology. In N. J. Lass, L. V. Reynolds, J. L. Northern, & D. E. Yoder (Eds.), *Handbook of Speech-Language Pathology and Audiology* (pp. 548–589). Toronto: B. C. Decker.

Thompson takes an appropriate critical stance toward current speech management procedures employed with childhood motor speech disorders. Her extensive review of the topic will clarify further what we know and do not know in speech habilitation of the child with neurologic impairment.

Feeding Therapy

Alexander, R. (1987a). Developing prespeech and feeding abilities in children. In S. Shanks (Ed.), *Nursing and the management of pediatric communication disorders*. San Diego, CA: College Hill Press.

Alexander, R. (1987b). Prespeech and feeding development. In E. McDonald (Ed.), *Treating cerebral palsy*. Austin, TX: Pro-ed.

Alexander, R. (1987c). Oral-motor treatment for infants and young children. *Seminars in Speech and Language, 8*, 87–100.

Morris, S. (1982). *The normal acquisitions of oral feeding skills: Implications for assessment and treatment.* Central Islip, NY: Therapeutic Media.

Morris, S. (1985). Developmental implications for the management of feeding problems in neurologically impaired children. *Seminars in Speech and Language, 6*, 293–315.

Morris, S. (1987). Therapy for the child with cerebral palsy: Interacting frameworks. *Seminars in Speech and Language, 8*, 71–86.

Morris, S., & Klien, M. D. (1987). *Prefeeding skills.* Tucson, AZ: Therapy Skill Builders.
Mueller, H. (1975). Feeding. In N. Finnie (Ed.), *Handling the young cerebral-palsied child at home* (2nd ed., pp. 113–132). New York: E. P. Dutton.

REFERENCES

Abbs, J. H., & Rosenbek, J. C. (1986). Some motor control perspectives on apraxia of speech and dysarthria. In J. M. Costello & A. Holland (Eds.), *Handbook of speech and language disorders* (pp. 371–407). San Diego: College Hill Press.

Alexander, R. (1987a). Prespeech and feeding development. In E. McDonald (Ed.), *Treating cerebral palsy.* Austin, TX: Pro-ed.

Alexander, R. (1987b). Oral-motor treatment for infants and young children with cerebral palsy. *Seminars in Speech and Language, 8,* 87–100.

Angelo, J. (1992). Comparison of three computer scanning modes as an interface method for persons with cerebral palsy. *American Journal of Occupational Therapy, 46,* 217–222.

Barlow, S. M., & Abbs, J. H. (1983). Force transducers for the evaluation of labial, lingual and mandibular function in dysarthria. *Journal of Speech and Hearing Research, 26,* 616–621.

Barlow, S. M., & Abbs, J. H. (1986). Fine force and position control of selected oral facial structures in upper motor neuron syndrome. *Experimental Neurology, 94,* 699–713.

Bax, M., & MacKeith, R. (1967). The results of treatment. *Developmental Medicine and Child Neurology, 9,* 1–2.

Bedrosian, J. L., Hoag, L. A., Johnson, D., & Calculator, S. (1998). Communicative competence as perceived by adults with severe speech impairments associated with cerebral palsy. *Journal of Speech, Language and Hearing Research, 41,* 667–675.

Bobath, B. (1967). Very early treatment of cerebral palsy. *Developmental Medicine and Child Neurology, 9,* 373–390.

Bobath, B. (1971). *Abnormal postural reflex activity caused by brain lesions.* London: Heinemann.

Bobath, K. (1980). *A neurophysiological basis for the treatment of cerebral palsy* (2nd ed.). Philadelphia: J. B. Lippencott.

Bobath, K., & Bobath, B. (1972). Cerebral palsy. In P. H. Pearson & C. E. Williams (Eds.), *Physical therapy services in the developmental disabilities.* Springfield, IL: Charles C. Thomas.

Brown, A. S., Silverman, J., Greenberg, S., Malamud, D. F., Album, M., Lloyd, R. W., & Sarshik, M. (1985). A team approach to drool control in cerebral palsy. *Annals of Plastic Surgery, 15,* 423–430.

Browne, D. (1966). Very early treatment of cerebral palsy. *Developmental Medicine and Child Neurology, 8,* 473.

Buzolich, M. J. (1987). Children in transition: Implementing augmentative communication systems with severely speech-handicapped children. *Seminars in Speech and Language, 8,* 199–213.

Cass, M. T. (1951). *Speech habilitation in cerebral palsy.* New York: Columbia University Press.

Culp, P. M. (1987). Outcome measurement: The impact of communication augmentation. *Seminars in Speech and Language, 8,* 169–181.

Dixon, C., & Curry, B. (1965). Some thoughts on the communication board. *Cerebral Palsy Journal, 26,* 12–15.

Dubner, R., Sessle, B. J., & Storey, A. T. (1978). *The neural basis of oral and facial function.* New York: Plenum.

Erenberg, G. (1984). Cerebral palsy. *Postgraduate Medicine, 75,* 87–93.

Feallock, B. (1958). Communication for the non-verbal individual. *American Journal of Occupational Therapy, 12,* 60–63, 83.

Ferry, P. C. (1981). On growing new neurons: Are early intervention programs effective? *Pediatrics, 67,* 38–41.

Goldberg, H. R., & Fenton, J. (n.d.). *Aphonic communication for those with cerebral palsy: Guide for the development of a conservation board.* New York: United Cerebral Palsy Association of New York.

Hardy, J. (1983). *Cerebral palsy.* Englewood Cliffs, NJ: Prentice Hall.

Hixon, T., & Hardy, J. (1964). Restricted motility of the speech articulators in cerebral palsy. *Journal of Speech and Hearing Disorders, 29,* 293–306.

Jaffe, M. B. (1986). Neurologic impairment of speech production: Assessment and treatment. In J. Costello & A. Holland (Eds.), *Handbook of speech and language disorders* (pp. 157–186). San Diego: College Hill Press.

Kates, B., & McNaughton, S. (1974). *The first application of Blissymbolics as a communication medium for the nonspeaking child: History and development 1971–1974.* Toronto: Blissymbolics Communication International.

Katona, F. (1989). Clinical neuro-developmental diagnosis and treatment. In P. R. Zelazo & R. G. Barr (Eds.), *Challenges to developmental paradigms: Implications for theory, assessment and treatment* (pp. 167–187). Hillsdale, NJ: Lawrence Erlbaum Associates.

Kong, E. (1966). Very early treatment of cerebral palsies. *Developmental Medicine and Child Neurology, 8,* 198–202.

Krusen, F., Kottke, F., & Ellwood, P. (1982). *Handbook of physical medicine and rehabilitation.* Philadelphia: W. B. Saunders.

Light, J. C., Binger, C., Agate, T. L., & Ramsay, K. N. (1999). Teaching partner-focused questions to individuals who use augmentative and alternative communication to enhance their communicative competence. *Journal of Speech, Language and Hearing Research, 42,* 241–255.

Light, J., Datillo, J., English, J., Guiterrez, L., & Hartz, J. (1992). Instructing facilitators to support the communication of people who use augmentative communication systems. *Journal of Speech and Hearing Research, 35,* 865–875.

Light, J., & Lindsay, P. (1992). Message encoding techniques for augmentative communication systems: The recall performance of adults with speech impairments. *Journal of Speech and Hearing Research, 35,* 853–864.

Lord, J. (1984). Cerebral palsy: A clinical approach. *Archives of Physical Medicine and Rehabilitation, 65,* 542–548.

Love, R. J., Hagerman, E. L., & Tiami, E. G. (1980). Speech performance, dysphagia, and oral reflexes in cerebral palsy. *Journal of Speech and Hearing Disorders, 45,* 59–75.

McDonald, E. T., & Chance, B., Jr. (1964). *Cerebral palsy.* Englewood Cliffs, NJ: Prentice-Hall.

McDonald, E. T., & Schutz, A. R. (1973). Communication boards for cerebral-palsied children. *Journal of Speech and Hearing Disorders, 38,* 73–88.

McNaughton, D., & Tawney, J. (1993). Comparison of two spelling instruction techniques for adults who use augmentative and alternative communication. *Augmentative and Alternate Communication, 9,* 72–82.

Montgomery, J. K. (1987). Augmentative communication: Selecting successful interventions. *Seminars in Speech and Language, 8,* 187–197.

Moore, C. A., & Ruark, J. L. (1996). Does speech emerge from earlier appearing oral motor behaviors? *Journal of Speech and Hearing Research, 39,* 1034–1047.

Morris, S. E. (1982). *Prespeech assessment scale: A rating scale for the measurement of prespeech behaviors from birth through two years.* Clifton, NJ: Preston.

Morris, S. E. (1985). Developmental implications for the management of feeding problems in neurologically impaired infants. *Seminars in Speech and Language, 6,* 293–315.

Morris, S. E. (1987). Therapy for children with cerebral palsy: Interacting frameworks. *Seminars in Speech and Language, 8,* 71–86.

Morris, S., & Klien, M. D. (1987). *Prefeeding skills.* Tucson, AZ: Therapy Skill Builders.

Musselwhite, C. R., & St. Louis, K. W. (1988). *Communication programming for persons with severe handicaps: Vocal and augmentative strategies* (2nd ed.). Boston: Little, Brown.

Neilson, P. D., & McCaughey, J. (1982). Self-regulation of spasm and spasticity in cerebral palsy. *Journal of Neurology, Neurosurgery and Psychiatry, 45,* 320–330.

Netsell, R., & Daniel, B. (1979). Dysarthria in adults: Physiologic approach to rehabilitation. *Archives of Physical Medicine & Rehabilitation, 60,* 502–508.

Netsell, R., Lotz, W. K., & Barlow, S. M. (1989). A speech physiology examination for individuals with dysarthria. In K. M. Yorkston & D. R. Beukelman (Eds.), *Recent advances in clinical dysarthria* (pp. 3–37). Boston: Little, Brown.

O'Dwyer, N. J., Neilson, P. D., Guitar, B., Quinn, P. T., & Andrews, G. (1983). Control of upper airway structures during nonspeech tasks in normal and cerebral-palsied subjects: EMG findings. *Journal of Speech and Hearing Research, 26,* 160–170.

Pearson, P. H. (1982). The results of treatment: The horns of our dilemma. *Developmental Medicine and Child Neurology, 24,* 417–418.

Richardson, S. A. (1972). People with cerebral palsy talk for themselves. *Developmental Medicine and Child Neurology, 14,* 525.

Russman, B. S., & Romnes, M. (1998). Neurorehabilitation for the child with cerebral palsy. In G. Miller & G. D. Clark (Eds.), *The cerebral palsies.* Boston: Butterworth-Heinemann.

Scherzer, A. L., Mike, V., & Ilson, J. (1976). Physical therapy as a determinant of change in the cerebral-palsied infant. *Pediatrics, 58,* 47–52.

Shane, H. (1987). Trends in communication aid technology for the severely speech-impaired. In W. Yule & M. Rutter (Eds.), *Language development and its disorders: Clinics in developmental medicine* (pp. 408–421). Philadelphia: Lippincott.

Shane, H. C., & Bashir, A. S. (1980). Election criteria for the adoption of an augmentative communications system: Preliminary considerations. *Journal of Speech and Hearing Disorders, 45,* 408–415.

Sheppard, J. J. (1964). Cranio-oropharyngeal motor patterns in dysarthria in cerebral palsy. *Journal of Speech and Hearing Research, 7,* 373–380.

Stark, R. E. (1985). Dysarthria in children. In J. G. Darby (Ed.), *Speech and language evaluation in neurology: Childhood disorders* (pp. 185–217). New York: Grune & Stratton.

Taft, L. T. (1972). Are we handicapping the handicapped? *Developmental Medicine and Child Neurology, 14,* 703–704.

Thompson, C. K. (1988). Articulation disorders in the child with neurogenic pathology. In N. J. Lass, L. V. McReynolds, J. L. Northern, & D. E. Yoder (Eds.), *Handbook of speech-language pathology and audiology* (pp. 548–591). Toronto: B. C. Decker.

Udwin, O. (1987). Analysis of the experimental adequacy of alternative communication training studies. *Child Language Teaching and Therapy, 3,* 18–29.

Vicker, B. (1974). *Nonoral communication systems project 1964/1972.* Iowa City: Campus Stores.

Westlake, H., & Rutherford, D. R. (1961). *Speech therapy for the cerebral-palsied.* Chicago: National Society for Crippled Children and Adults.

Wilkie, T. F. (1967). The problem of drooling in cerebral palsy: A surgical approach. *Canadian Journal of Surgery, 10,* 60–65.

Wilkie, T. F., & Brody, G. S. (1977). The surgical treatment of drooling—A ten year review. *Plastic and Reconstructive Surgery, 58,* 791–800.

Woolridge, C. P., & Russell, G. (1976). Head position training with the cerebral-palsied child: Application of biofeedback techniques. *Archives of Physical Medicine and Rehabilitation, 57,* 407–414.

Wright, T., & Nicholson, J. (1973). Physiotherapy for the spastic child: Evaluation. *Developmental Medicine and Child Neurology, 15,* 146–163.

Yorkston, K. M. (1996). Treatment efficacy: Dysarthria. *Journal of Speech and Hearing Research, 5,* 546–557.

Yorkston, K. M., Beukelman, D. R., & Bell, K. R. (1986). *Clinical management of dysarthric speakers.* Boston: Little, Brown.

► # 8

Therapy for Childhood Motor Speech Disability

*The approach emphasizes the component-by-component
analysis of the peripheral speech mechanism, where
the selection and sequence of treatment procedures
follow from the physiologic nature and severity
of involvement in each component.*
—RONALD NETSELL AND BILLIE DANIEL, 1979

*A Subsystems Approach to the Management of the
Childhood Dysarthrias*

Respiratory Dysfunction
  Seating for Adequate Respiratory Performance • Expanding Physiological
  Breath Support for Speech • Speaking Within Respiratory Limits •
  Speech Phrasing

Laryngeal Dysfunction
  Hypo- and Hyperfunctional Voice Symptoms • Adolescent Voice
  Management • Loudness Symptoms • Pitch and Stress Symptoms

Velopharyngeal Dysfunction
  Netsell's Contribution • Palatal Exercises • Pharyngeal Flap Surgery •
  Palatal Lift Prosthesis • Traditional Methods of Resource Management

Articulatory Muscle Dysfunction
  Opposing Approaches • Guidelines for Selection of Target Sounds •
  Articulation Management Guidelines • Neurologic Symptoms in

A SUBSYSTEMS APPROACH TO THE MANAGEMENT OF THE CHILDHOOD DYSARTHRIAS

A subsystems approach to the analysis and management of the dysarthrias of childhood has actually been long accepted in the field of clinical speech neurology (Froeschels, 1952; McDonald & Chance, 1964; Westlake & Rutherford, 1961). Current approaches to the analysis and treatment of the childhood dysarthrias are based on this early literature as well as more current reports of the use of the subsystems approach with adult dysarthrias. These more recent approaches are reflected in the work of Barlow (1989); Barlow and Farley (1989); Darley, Aronson, and Brown (1975); Hardy (1983); Netsell, Lotz, and Barlow (1989); and Yorkston, Beukelman, and Bell (1986). Although current laboratory approaches reflected in recent work appear promising for the treatment of childhood dysarthrias, these sophisticated speech laboratories are not always available to the clinician in the field. In this chapter, suggestions for management assume that a well-equipped speech science laboratory is not readily available. It should be pointed out that a laboratory approach is not always necessary for the management of every dysarthric child. It is appropriate only for an age-limited population of children (Thompson, 1988).

Some infants and young children with neurologic impairment do not have the maturity to participate fully in a subsystems approach to assessment and therapy. Moreover, currently there is scant research evidence of the positive effects of a subsystems therapy approach on children. In general, the speech-language pathologist is still forced to rely on the limited evidence from case studies of successfully treated adult dysarthrics and the observations of experienced clinicians to support the rationale of most management programs used with child dysarthrics.

This lack of documentation of what may be called the traditional speech subsystems approach to therapy has led some speech-language pathologists to elect, and depend heavily on, alternate and augmentative communication aid devices, even in very young children, without attempting a concentrated program of oral speech development (Musselwhite & St. Louis, 1988). Advocates of a speech subsystems approach in dysarthria have usually set as a primary goal the production and use of the best oral speech that the child is capable of using within the physical limitations of the neurologic impairment. Augmentative communicative aids generally play a secondary role to oral speech habilitation in a subsystems approach unless it is abundantly clear that the child has little potential for speech development (Hardy, 1983; Lotz & Netsell, 1989; Yorkston et al., 1986). If the child has little potential for oral speech, communication aid technology can be employed successfully in most cases (see Chapter 7).

A subsystems therapeutic approach to speech management generally recognizes the five broad functional components of the speech process with which the speech pathologist must deal in evaluation and therapy: (1) respiration, (2) phonation, (3) articulation, (4) resonation, and (5) prosody. Netsell and Daniel (1979) in addition have listed 10 functional structures that are critically important in evaluation and therapy of these processes. These structures are

1. abdominal muscles,
2. diaphragm,
3. rib cage,
4. larynx,
5. tongue/pharynx,
6. posterior tongue,
7. anterior tongue,
8. velopharynx,
9. jaw, and
10. lips.

They also list a series of aerodynamic measures of the vocal tract that allow the speech-language pathologist to diagnose malfunctioning of the various muscular valving systems in the vocal tract. These aerodynamic measures include: (1) subglottal air pressure, (2) intraoral air pressure, (3) glottal air flow, (4) oral air flow, and (5) nasal air flow. Speech management in the childhood dysarthrias must aim to improve the muscular functioning involved with the 10 functional structures of the vocal tract that generate or valve the airstream for speech. Appropriate management techniques should attempt to normalize the two pressure measures and three air flow measures as much as possible. Netsell and Daniel (1979) point out that very different techniques may be needed to improve the functioning within each of the broad components of respiration, phonation, articulation, resonation, and prosody.

RESPIRATORY DYSFUNCTION

There is considerable agreement among speech experts that the dysarthric child with either UMN or LMN lesions may present breathing disturbances that result in disrupted speech performance. There is much less agreement among these same experts, however, on what therapeutic procedures are most effective in modifying these breathing abnormalities. Hardy (1964) not only has researched the problem more carefully than has any other student of childhood dysarthria but also has presented the most thoughtful approach to management of respiratory dysfunction. His view of breathing management in the childhood dysarthrias is relied upon heavily (Hardy, 1964, 1983; Hardy & Edmonds, 1968).

Seating for Adequate Respiratory Performance

As a preliminary to respiration therapy, it is necessary for the speech-language pathologist to ensure that the child is adequately positioned for speaking. Since unsupported sitting with adequate head control and good posture is often delayed in children with motor impairment, it is not uncommon to find dysarthric children sitting without adequate upright support or with poor postural support provided by pillows, belts, or canvas strollers. It is critical that the child be provided with appropriate support that results in normal neck elongation and head and shoulder alignment as well as firm trunk support and stability of the spine. The most appropriate position is a seated posture in which the function of the upper extremities, head control, eye contact, and vocalization are enhanced. The child's pelvis is in a neutral position so that he is sitting on the ischial tuberosities as opposed to the sacrum. Hips should be flexed and slightly abducted. A seat belt may be used to secure the pelvis in a correct position in the child's chair. The seat of the chair is manipulated to provide an angle of less than 90° between the back of the chair and the seat. This prevents the child from arching out of the chair during body extension (Porter, Wurth, & Stowers, 1988). Side supports are used to correct scoliosis and to keep the trunk as symmetrical as possible. Strapping systems are sometimes employed to control kyphosis or lordosis. Although some experts have argued that an upright sitting position is not always conducive to respiratory support for phonation, Hardy (1983) believes that in the cerebral-palsied dysarthric child, respiratory support does not usually vary significantly in either supine, prone, or sitting positions. Yorkston et al. (1986), however, note that the supine position sometimes enhances phonation in adult dysarthrics over other positions, and Putnam and Hixon (1984) have pointed out that where muscle weakness is a large component of the neurologic impairment, the effect of position may play a highly significant role in breath support. Therefore, testing the child's individual ability to generate adequate breath support in various positions is important.

Expanding Physiological Breath Support for Speech

Westlake and Rutherford (1961) introduced the concept of working beyond minimal motor requirements in training the speech mechanism of dysarthrics.

In other words, they argued for increasing physiologic support for speech. Canter (1965) provided a rationale for training physiologic support for breath control before speech production is begun. It is my belief that significant changes in physiological support for speech in children cannot always be made by employing the traditional respiratory training techniques of the average speech therapy room. Only in rare instances have I seen respiratory capacity significantly modified with subsequent positive results in speech breathing. In one instance, a child with moderately severe cerebral palsy was introduced into a swimming class and mastered the Australian crawl and the breathing pattern associated with that stroke. In another instance an adolescent cerebral-palsied child took part in a free-weight training program that strengthened and developed his upper body. In both instances significant gains in muscle strength and control of respiratory muscles improved speech performance. These are unusual cases, however, in which more effective means were employed than are usually available in the average therapy room.

Although dramatic changes in respiratory abilities as those just described may not be expected in every child, phonatory drills requiring maximal levels of performance are not always unwarranted activities in the therapy room. These drills provide practice in using phonatory skills for expanding physiological support for speech acts. This may be very important for the dysarthric child in speaking situations that demand she or he go beyond the usual functional limits of her or his respiratory-laryngeal system. This may be particularly critical in the mildly motor-involved child whose speech performance must be competitive or near competitive with the normal-speaking child in our society.

Speaking Within Respiratory Limits

The unlikelihood of making dramatic changes in respiratory capacities in the usual speech-therapy situations highlights the belief that speech skills must be trained within the child's respiratory limits (Hardy, 1983). Thompson (1988) has documented several techniques for modifying speech skills within the respiratory limits of the child. She trains, as the first order of business, the child's capacity to increase air intake. Using the child's mean duration of inhalation as a guide, she sets a target of inspiratory duration for the child and instructs him in deep inhalation. On-going feedback is provided. For instance, the child's hand may be placed on the epigastrium to monitor the movement of the rib cage and abdomen in attempts to control the inhalation process. A dry spirometer may be employed to provide feedback of improving inspiration. Using the full face mask of a wet spirometer is generally contraindicated. It may disrupt the natural respiratory behavior of the child and does not afford appropriate feedback in young and unsophisticated children.

Next, phonation production must be introduced, usually in the form of producing a sustained vowel. This activity brings to the child's awareness the expiratory phase of respiration. Inhaling to relatively high lung-volume levels and phonating before a mirror alerts the child to the relationship between the inspiratory and expiratory processes in speech as the thoracic and abdominal respiratory patterns are observed. Hardy (1983) provides descriptions of several techniques for training a child in awareness of this relationship. Using a pencil or a crayon to illustrate the short duration of inhalation and extended duration of exhalation in the child's actual phonation attempts is probably one of the more effective methods for training patterns of speech breathing.

In the past, sustained blowing, as opposed to sustained phonation, was often used as a method to train exhalation. This training technique is probably contraindicated in most cases since, as yet, there is no solid research evidence that blowing increases the expiratory phase of breathing for speech. In fact, vocal tract valving for blowing and speech are quite different. In speech and vowel phonation, velopharyngeal activity in particular is different than it is in blowing. Tongue and lip valving is also obviously different in speech and blowing activities. Although blowing may increase respiratory and laryngeal motor control in general, it is unlike the motor control necessary for prolonged breath support for speech.

As noted earlier, Hardy (1983) has indicated that improved vocal and speech performance results when there are relatively high levels of lung volume to support the performance. However, Hardy does not recommend that the child be instructed to take a maximal deep breath before speaking. Rather, he believes that the best strategy for developing adequately high levels of lung volume is to put off training until the child is producing connected speech routinely. At this point in training, the child naturally requires adequate speech breath support and will develop it to a degree that will support her language use in consonant-vowel combination, syllables, and words as well as in word combinations and phases.

In some cases, it may be very difficult to extend the levels of lung volume to support the speech performance of which the child is capable. Some children may circumvent this problem by improving the use of breath control by other means. Improvement of articulation production usually allows better valving of the airstream for speech with more efficient use of available air. Use of a palatal lift prosthesis or a pharyngeal flap in a child with a nasal air leak resulting from a paralyzed or uncoordinated soft palate will also improve valving and use of intraoral air during speech.

Measurement of breath support and increasing expiratory control is mandatory in a well-organized therapy plan (Thompson, 1988). Hixon, Hawley, and Wilson (1982) have described a homemade device, pictured in Figure 8-1, constructed from a water glass, straw, and paper clip that allows the speech pathologist to estimate respiratory driving pressure (subglottal air pressure). As a rule of thumb, the ability to generate subglottic pressure

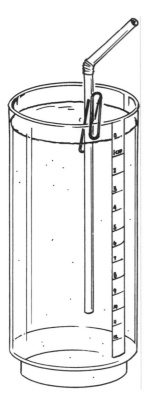

FIGURE 8-1   A Homemade Device for the Clinical Estimation of Respiratory Driving Pressure in Child Dysarthrics

From "An around-the-house device for the clinical determination of respiratory driving pressure: A note on making simple even simpler" by T. Hixon, J. Hawley, and J. Wilson, 1982, *Journal of Speech and Hearing Disorders, 47,* p. 413.

within a range of 5 to 10 cm of water for more than a duration of 5 seconds approximates normal adult ranges of control (Rosenbek & LaPointe, 1985). Data for normal children is not available on this task, to my knowledge. A slightly more sophisticated device for establishing pressure measures is an oral manometer with a leak valve. Oral manometers are moderately expensive and are usually readily available at a local medical supply house. These instruments are useful when there is no access to a well-outfitted speech science laboratory. Other more elaborate respiratory measurement devices often found in clinical laboratories are discussed in Yorkston et al. (1986).

Speech Phrasing

A time-honored and effective technique for controlling respiratory air flow during speaking is the use of speech phrasing. The goal is to produce short patterns of utterance between more-frequent-than-normal inspirations. The use of short utterances with well-timed inhalations between phrases usually allows the dysarthric child to communicate without the loss of intelligibility that may occur when a speaker attempts to articulate speech without sufficient breath support. Careful attention must be given to training the dysarthric child so that he clearly understands the goal and mechanisms of speech phrasing. Some older children may reject phrasing as a reasonable training technique because they realize that their present dysarthric speech is slower than normal and they fear speech phrasing will slow it even further. The older child is usually fully aware that a slowed rate of speech is viewed as a negative aspect of dysarthric speech by some listeners. In fact, it is usually a particularly salient negative feature in the public mind and often serves as a significant socially stigmatizing aspect of motor disability. If the dysarthric child, however, can be convinced that slowed and phrased speech will yield a considerable gain in overall intelligibility, she will frequently accept the idea that the technique is important to her image as an effective communicator.

Even if the communicative attempt is only a series of simple word approximations, the child must be taught to judge how many words can be uttered on one breath group. In young and/or severely involved children, even multisyllable words may have to be produced on more than one expiration to achieve adequate intelligibility (Hardy, 1983).

Most children easily learn the logic of simple phrase divisions and can be taught to recognize a phrase unit if the clinician provides examples they can hear and imitate. Older children, who can read and who have the appropriate language capacity to utter grammatically complex material, will benefit from seeing a printed transcript of their speech to determine what is a manageable phrase length. If they actually use a pencil to mark phrase limits and then read and rehearse this transcript as if it were a speech to be recorded electronically or delivered to an audience, they usually begin to see the benefits of the concept of speech phrasing. Listening to their tape-recorded efforts to phrase usually helps convince dysarthrics that there is considerable gain in speech intelligibility when speech is appropriately phrased.

Phrasing and slowing the speech rate may also be accomplished by using a pacing board with dysarthric children. Developed by Helm (1979), the pacing board shown in Figure 8-2 consists of a slotted board with each slot given a different color. The dysarthric child may be asked to touch one slot per word or one slot per short phrase. The technique serves to meter the speech and separates each word or phrase in an utterance.

LARYNGEAL DYSFUNCTION

Hypo- and Hyperfunctional Voice Symptoms

Laryngeal symptoms associated with neurologic impairment have been described often, but systematic approaches for modifying these symptoms have been poorly documented. Most authorities have been very cautious about asserting that vocal symptoms can be relieved with therapy. Aronson

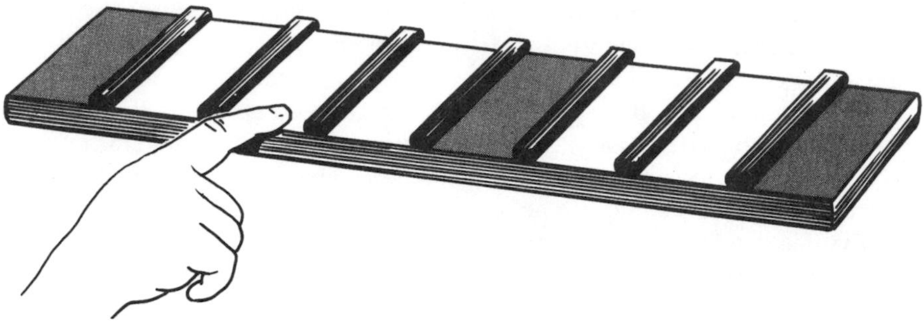

FIGURE 8-2   A Pacing Board

From "Management of palilalia with a pacing board" by N. A. Helm, 1979, *Journal of Speech and Hearing Disorders, 44*, pp. 350–353.

(1985), speaking of adult dysarthria, says, ". . . most voice disorders due to nervous system diseases are resistant to modification" (p. 153). Hardy (1983) observes that vocal dysfunction in cerebral palsy may range from a complete inability to adduct the vocal folds to the more common type of vocal dysfunction in which there appears to be extreme degrees of physiologic effort or hyperfunction. In some cases the dysarthric child can do little more than produce an undifferentiated vowel. At best this hyperfunctional voice yields a very strained voice quality. For all these situations Hardy suggests a negative prognosis generally, but he does recommend a trial period of management with apparently little hope of improvement for most cases.

Adolescent Voice Management

In less severe cases of hyperfunctional laryngeal involvement in which the child displays deviant, but not dysphonic, phonation, I have found that a trial of voice intervention to modify deviant pitch and loudness can sometimes bring surprising results. At one point in our ongoing program for child dysarthrics with cerebral palsy, we introduced a small group of adolescent children to therapy in an attempt to modify pitch and loudness. We attribute success in this area to the fact that these children, who had had speech training almost all of their lives, had never been exposed to any direct voice training procedures during their long years of therapy. As preschoolers and elementary-school children, most had been given intensive oral muscle training in preparation for articulation training. Articulation training was intensive with emphasis usually on phonetic placement. When the child had attained a moderate degree of intelligibility for communication purposes, the major goal of therapy was thought to have been attained. These children rarely had been given the opportunity to listen to their own voices on tape recorders and had little chance to practice traditional vocal training techniques. We specifically employed auditory training techniques in which the child is asked to identify and discriminate among the various types of vocal productions made in terms of loudness, pitch, and quality dimensions. Our dysarthric children had neither been required to try to match a variety of vocal dimensions produced by their clinicians nor had they been given training in listening to their own voices or in attempting to modify them with the use of a tape recorder.

This is not to say that all dysarthric children will be able to modify their vocal symptoms by traditional auditory training methods of voice therapy, but with effort some will be able to produce voice with more ease and normality. The result will be increased intelligibility and a reduction in socially stigmatizing vocal symptoms. The voices of most child dysarthics, even with training, usually lack the normal flexibility of pitch, loudness, and quality seen in normal children. Even in the child whose primary mode of communication will be an augmentative device, improvement in articulation and voice will help speed the whole communicative interaction.

Loudness Symptoms

Loudness dimensions are generally more easily modified than are other dimensions of voice in child dysarthrics. Muscle weakness, commonly associated with LMN disorders but sometimes present in UMN disorders, also is generally associated with a soft and breathy voice. Hypoadduction of the voice is assumed in these cases. Fiberoptic techniques for viewing the larynx in childhood dysarthrics have not yet been reported, so there is no objective evidence of flaccid vocal folds as yet in LMN disorders. However, the soft, breathy voice associated with substantial muscle weakness may be modified by exercises that increase vocal effort. An often recommended technique for increasing the tonus of the laryngeal musculature is the use of "pushing" procedures (Froeschels, Kastein, & Weiss, 1955). The child is asked to grasp a rod at chest height or to hold the edges of a chair and push hard. Increased tonus produced by muscle contraction during pushing is often associated with increased tonus in the laryngeal muscles. Thompson (1988) has noted that if there is general body weakness, this exercise may be ineffective since the motor weakness problem may be too pervasive to generate needed tone in the vocal folds. If tonus in the laryngeal area cannot be sufficiently increased, portable vocal amplifiers may be considered as augmentative aids (Yorkston et al., 1986).

Hardy (1983) has observed that the use of a palatal lift prosthesis, ostensibly to improve velopharyngeal dysfunction, may improve the valving of the total vocal tract, reducing air escapage at critical valving points and normalizing loudness in flaccid dysarthrics. Management for velopharyngeal problems that cause air wastage and weak voice in spastic children is usually deferred in the time sequence of activities of the management program. Developing feeding and oral-motor skills, rudimentary language, and functional articulation skills often is given early priority in therapy. When problems of hypernasality and soft breathy voice symptoms emerge in the child's utterances, then velopharyngeal management should be considered in these children. The use of a palatal lift does not always produce immediate success in reducing hypernasality or air wastage with loudness problems (Lotz & Netsell, 1989).

Pitch and Stress Symptoms

Treatment for pitch deviations in childhood dysarthria usually centers on three goals: (1) lower pitch, (2) raise pitch, and (3) increase pitch flexibility. Auditory and visual biofeedback is helpful in allowing the child to monitor his attempts to modify pitch. Thompson (1988) has recommended the use of a commercial instrument, *Visipitch* (Kay Elemetrics Corp.), to help the child in these efforts. The tape recorder has been used successfully as a pitch (and loudness) monitoring device for several years and is still very useful. Variation in intonation should be taught to increase pitch flexibility. Diagramming rising and failing pitch contours in syllables, words, and phrases has proved helpful with several children.

Yorkston et al. (1986) emphasize the need for dysarthric speakers to learn to identify targeted linguistic stress in a breath group and then to signal that stress appropriately in their speaking attempts. Attention to stress patterns and their appropriate monitoring in spontaneous speech tends to maximize speech naturalness in the dysarthric person. These activities are generally more appropriate for the older child since they involve advanced perceptual and cognitive skills. There is little evidence of their effectiveness in a younger child population as yet.

VELOPHARYNGEAL DYSFUNCTION

Netsell's Contribution

Netsell (1969) deserves credit for bringing to the attention of workers in the field of childhood dysarthria the fact that velopharyngeal dysfunction is often a major aspect of the speech problem in dysarthria. His documentation of the several ways in which velopharyngeal functioning can be disturbed in cerebral palsy clarified the important role that the velopharynx plays in defective speech (see Chapter 3). Since his seminal 1969 article appeared, considerable study of the remediation of velopharyngeal defects, both in children and adults, has been reported. Because velopharyngeal problems are to a degree similar in both the dysarthric and cleft palate child, it is possible to draw conclusions from the literature of velopharyngeal management in craniofacial anomalies and apply them with caution to the management of childhood dysarthrics. Three basic approaches have been described for remediation of velopharyngeal dysfunctioning in both categories of children. They are (1) palatal exercises, (2) palatal prosthesis in the form of a palatal lift, and (3) pharyngeal flap surgery.

Palatal Exercises

Of the three remediation approaches, palatal exercises appears to be the most controversial. There has been no published evidence to my knowledge that palatal exercise is effective in cerebral-palsied children. Reports of the effectiveness of palatal exercise to remediate hypernasality in children with LMN disorders are also unavailable.

Two common exercise approaches have been suggested: massage of the soft palate and pushing exercises. To perform palatal massage, the speech pathologist is instructed to place a finger cot on the finger and gently massage the child's velum in a posterior to anterior direction. This is said to stimulate sensation and to activate muscle contraction; it also has been suggested that an artist's paint brush may be used to stimulate movement (Cole, 1971). Further, it appears critical that the child learn to observe in a mirror the movement of the soft palate during the massage and stimulation process. The child should be encouraged to duplicate at a voluntary level palatal movements brought about by external stimulation and massage, according to Cole.

Froeschels et al. (1955) have indicated that pushing exercises, described earlier, can be effective for velar paralysis. As large muscle groups are voluntarily contracted during pushing exercises, muscle overflow may occur in the palatopharyngeal muscles and aid velopharyngeal closure.

Palatal exercise has been studied widely in cleft palate children (Ruscello, 1982). Ruscello's review of the research indicates that palatal exercise techniques are not universally successful in the cleft palate population or the normal population. Best results appear to occur when children know what levels of elevation their palates have reached. With neuromuscular paralysis or incoordination, the results are likely to be even less successful than in cleft palate children. The technique of palatal exercise therefore must be considered only experimental in the dysarthric population.

Pharyngeal Flap Surgery

A technique that has been highly successful in reducing problems of hypernasality in cleft palate children has been pharyngeal flap surgery. The plastic surgeon raises a flap of muscular tissue from the posterior pharyngeal wall and inserts it into the velum. On contraction of velopharyngeal muscles, the tissue of the flap acts as a muscular "plug" to close the velopharyngeal opening and reduce nasal resonance. The effectiveness of the procedure with craniofacial anomalies prompted speech-language pathologists to test its value with dysarthric children. As early as 1961, Hardy, Rembolt, Spriesterbach, and Jaypathy reported the results of pharyngeal flap surgery with three cerebral-palsied children. The two older children, both older than 10 years of age, showed good speech gains in velopharyngeal closure, and the younger child was able to obtain increased intraoral breath pressure. In 1983, however, Hardy expressed the opinion that results from pharyngeal flap surgery were disappointing in dysarthric children, and he reported that he was now recommending a palatal lift prosthesis for children with neurologic impairment. Others have considered a pharyngeal flap only if a palatal lift prosthesis fails in cerebral-palsied children (Lotz & Netsell, 1989).

Our experience has been that plastic surgeons are often reluctant to perform palatopharyngeal surgery on dysarthric children. They believe that paralyzed palatopharyngeal muscles predispose the results of the surgical procedure to failure or partial success. At present, pharyngeal flap surgery remains a treatment of second choice in childhood dysarthria (Hardy, 1983; Lotz & Netsell, 1989; Salomonson, Kawamoto, & Wilson, 1988).

Palatal Lift Prosthesis

The palatal lift prosthesis, as shown in Figure 8-3, appears to be the most viable management approach available when hypernasality is a hazard to speech intelligibility in childhood dysarthria. The palatal lift prosthesis has several advantages for the improvement of speech intelligibility in childhood dysarthria (Hardy, 1983). First, it allows the child to develop and maintain sufficient intraoral air pressure to produce consonantal sounds more normally. Second, the aerodynamic aspects of the vocal tract are improved so that there is an increase in the duration of utterances on one expiration. This permits an increased vocal output. Third, it has been observed that tongue postures for vowel production become more normal after placement of the prosthesis. Fourth, the palatal lift allows more normal velopharyngeal closure to occur, thus reducing the threat that hypernasality offers to speech intelligibility.

Although palatal lift prosthesis is thought of primarily as a measure to reduce hypernasality, Hardy (1983) is of the opinion that the reduced intraoral pressure of hypernasality is often a relatively minor problem in the speech of dysarthric speakers compared to the major effect that velopharyngeal incompetence has upon the aerodynamic and mechanical aspects of the vocal mechanism. Loudness symptoms are improved.

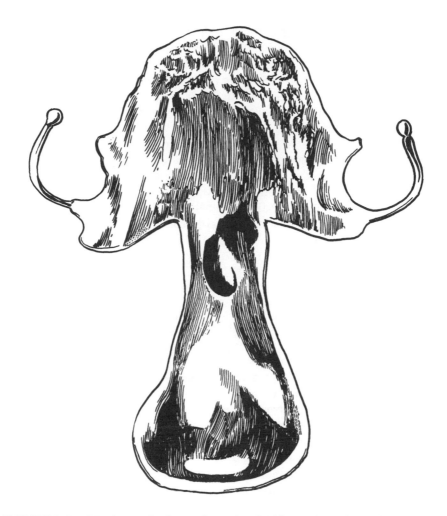

FIGURE 8-3   Horizontal View of a Palatal Lift Designed to Elevate the Soft Palate

From "Palatal lift prosthesis for the treatment of palatopharyngeal incompetency" by W. E. LaVelle and J. C. Hardy, 1979, *Journal of Prosthetic Dentistry, 42,* p. 308.

There are, however, some contraindications to the use of a palatal lift prosthesis in a dysarthric child. First, if the speech musculature is severely motor involved, it is highly likely that the speech will remain unintelligible even with reduced hypernasality. Second, the child with UMN lesions and a hyperactive gag reflex may find it difficult to be fitted with a palatal lift prosthesis and may have difficulty tolerating it over time. Third, motor involvement may preclude independent insertion, removal, and cleansing of the prosthesis.

If initial fitting of a palatal lift prosthesis can be tolerated by the dysarthric child, it usually becomes a very effective aid because the velar portion of the lift can be reshaped after the first fitting to provide comfort and maximum effectiveness over time. It is critical that the speech-language pathologist and prosthodontist cooperate closely in the fitting of the prosthesis. It is important that the speech-language pathologist be available to decide if the hypernasality has been reduced adequately and to make sure that the velar portion of the prosthesis is not producing elements of hyponasality. The speech-language pathologist is in the best position of all professionals to refer the child to the prosthodontist for further adjustments.

Fitting of a palatal lift prosthesis may afford some difficult problems in dysarthric children. Lotz and Netsell (1989) have described an attempt to fit such a prosthesis in a 12-year-old cerebral-palsied child. Sensory loss and an uncomfortable fit made the use of the palatal lift prosthesis very difficult. The recommendation of pharyngeal flap surgery finally was made in this case.

Traditional Methods of Resonance Management

More traditional methods of remediation to improve nasal resonance may be used for individuals with cases of mild hypernasality who are not being considered for a palatal lift prosthesis or pharyngeal flap surgery. Auditory discrimination procedures to teach the child to detect the presence or absence of hypernasality in her own voice are helpful. Hardy (1983) recommends the use of a dental mirror below the nostrils to visualize nasal air emission or the use of visual feedback to demonstrate nasal escapage to the child. Feathers, tissue paper, or other light objects held below the nostrils of the child are helpful here.

Use of blowing techniques to improve velopharyngeal closure and occlusion of the nostrils to produce speech without abnormality is generally to be discouraged (McWilliams, Morris, & Shelton, 1990), since blowing activities call for types of palatopharyngeal movement that are unlike movements used in speaking. Occlusion of the nostrils is said to create "palatal surrender," a situation in which the child may not use the soft palate in velopharyngeal closure activities as it should be used. In summary, there is increasing attention given to velopharyngeal dysfunction in child dysarthrics. Speech pathologists must recognize that several options are available for management.

ARTICULATORY MUSCLE DYSFUNCTION

Opposing Approaches

It has been traditional in the treatment of childhood dysarthria to provide articulation therapy as a major component of a speech management program.

Management plans of the past often included a regime of oral exercise to improve strength, agility, and range of motion of lips, tongue, and jaw as a prerequisite to articulation therapy. Therapists who felt that nonspeech exercises were irrelevant often began articulation therapy directly. In both approaches, articulation therapy acted as the royal road to improved intelligibility of speech in childhood dysarthria. Those speech-language pathologists who preceded articulation therapy with oral exercises often moved directly to a phonetic placement approach for the development and remediation of speech sounds. This approach was supported by the logic that oral exercise programs would bring to the child's awareness the concepts of speech movement patterns, focal articulation points, and use of adequate force and appropriate range of movement to produce speech.

On the other hand, those who did not use oral exercises and phonetic placement stressed the need to group vowel and consonant articulation errors into logical sets and then simultaneously correct as many of these error sounds as possible without confusing the child (Hardy, 1983). Hardy stresses the need to move as quickly as possible from training CV syllables to training speech sounds in words and syllables. Hardy notes that visual feedback for speech is appropriate for some children and not others. He holds that instructions that draw specific attention to certain structures and movements, as in phonetic placement approaches, make voluntary articulation production very difficult for some children. Although clearly two distinct approaches to train articulation in dysarthric children exist, no data is yet available as to the effectiveness of either approach.

Guidelines for Selection of Target Sounds

Despite the lack of data to support different approaches to articulation treatment, some guidelines seem reasonable in planning a therapy program (Thompson, 1988). Thompson suggests that target sounds for correction be chosen by careful diagnostic articulation testing. Although several articulation tests are appropriate for the task, I suggest using the *Fisher-Logemann Test of Articulation Competence* (1971), shown in Figure 8-4, initially. It provides an excellent display of place and manner errors, as well as voicing errors, as they appear in prevocalic, intervocalic, and postvocalic positions.

After a detailed articulation analysis using narrow transcription, Thompson chooses specific targets for treatment. Guidelines for target selection include:

1. Errors that are stimulable are chosen over those that are not.
2. Sounds that are produced correctly in one position are chosen over those that are never produced correctly in any position.
3. Distorted sounds are usually corrected before sound substitutions or sound omissions.
4. More visible sounds are chosen over those that are less visible.

THE FISHER-LOGEMANN TEST OF ARTICULATION COMPETENCE

Screening ☐ Complete ☐

Record Form for the Picture Test

Name_____ Date_____ Examiner_____

Age_____ Grade (or Occupation)_____ School (or Employer)_____

Birthdate_____ Home Address_____

Native Dialect_____ Foreign Language in home_____

CONSONANT PHONEMES

Card #	IPA Phoneme	Common Spelling	Dev. Age	Place of Articulation	Voicing	Stop Pre.	Stop Inter.	Stop Post.	Fricative Pre.	Fricative Inter.	Fricative Post.	Affricate Pre.	Affricate Inter.	Affricate Post.	Glide Pre.	Glide Inter.	Glide Post.	Lateral Pre.	Lateral Inter.	Lateral Post.	Nasal Pre.	Nasal Inter.	Nasal Post.
1	p	p	3	Bilabial	Ʉ	/p	/p	/p	/ʍ¹														
2	b	b	5																				
3	ʍ	wh	3																				
4	w	w			V	/b	/b	/b							/w	/w							
5	m	m	3																	/m	/m	/m
6	f	f	4	Labio-dental	Ʉ				/f	/f	/f												
7	v	v	7		V				/v	/v	/v												
8	θ	th	7	Tip-dental	Ʉ				/θ	/θ	/θ												
9	ð	th	8		V				/ð	/ð	/ð												
10	t	t	6	Tip-alveolar	Ʉ	/t	/t²	/t															
11	d	d	5																				
12	l	l	6															/l	/l	/l			
13	n	n	3		V	/d	/d	/d													/n	/n	/n
14	s	s	7	Blade-alveolar	Ʉ				/s	/s	/s												
15	z	z	7		V				/z	/z	/z												
16	ʃ	sh	6	Blade-prepalatal	Ʉ				/ʃ	/ʃ	/ʃ	/tʃ	/tʃ	/tʃ									
17	ʒ	zh	7																				
18	tʃ	ch	6		V							/ʒ	/ʒ³	/dʒ	/dʒ	/dʒ							
19	dʒ	j	7																				
20	j	y	5	Front-palatal	Ʉ																		
					V										/j	/j							
21	r	r	6	Central-palatal	Ʉ																		
					V										/r	/r	/r⁴						
22	k	k	4	Back-velar	Ʉ	/k	/k	/k															
23	g	g	4																				
24	ŋ	ng	5		V	/g	/g	/g													/ŋ	/ŋ	
25	h	h	3	Glottal	Ʉ				/h	/h													

SUMMARY OF MISARTICULATION PATTERNS:

MANNER OF FORMATION ERRORS:

PLACE OF ARTICULATION ERRORS:

VOICING ERRORS:

Notes: (These and additional notes are discussed in the Manual under "Dialectal Variations")
1. Either /ʍ/ or /w/   3. Either /ʒ/ or /dʒ/.
2. Either /t/ or /d/   4. Either /r/ or /ə/ or lengthening of the preceding vowel.

FIGURE 8-4 Test Useful for Phonetic Analysis in Childhood Dysarthria

Source: Fisher, H.B., & Logemann, J.A. (1971). *Fisher-Logemann Test of Articulation Competence.* Austin, TX: Pro-ed. Reprinted by permission.

5. Early-developing sounds are chosen over late-developing sounds. In addition, sounds in a particular place, manner, voicing category, or phonologic process category may be selected.

Crary and Comeau (1981) advocate identification and intervention programs for congenital dysarthrics based on the assessment of general phonological processes in the dysarthric speech pattern. Documenting this approach with a 25-year-old spastic cerebral-palsied female, they indicate improved intelligibility of speech after a training program directed at the phonological processes errors in the subject's speech. They found that this subject primarily demonstrated cluster and stopping errors in her speech pattern. Reduction of cluster complexity included replacing fricatives with homorganic stops, deleting final consonants, and voicing prevocalic voiceless stops. Therapy was aimed at modifying the stopping process, which was the most frequent problem. The results of the program indicated a reduction in the frequency of the stopping processes, which produced an increase in correct fricatives in spontaneous speech.

More data on the effectiveness of therapy employing the phonologic process approach in child dysarthria is needed. The study by Crary and Comeau suggests a possible alternate approach to more traditional articulation therapy for childhood dysarthria, but its effectiveness has not been reported beyond this single case.

Articulation Management Guidelines

Based on his wide experience with childhood dysarthria, Hardy (1983) has offered several guidelines for the management of articulatory errors. Among the procedures he advocates are

1. training consonant errors that are produced correctly in prevocalic positions but are misarticulated in postvocalic positions; postvocalic position errors will be remediated more easily after the phoneme has been established in the prevocalic position.
2. intensive training of articulatory distortions that fall short of target articulation points because of obvious motor involvement; in such cases, the prognosis for achieving focal contacts is usually good.
3. referred training in articulatory omissions and distortions that are based on obvious motor involvement, since these are generally more difficult to improve until articulatory distortions are reversed.
4. using a multiple auditory-visual stimulation (look-listen) approach rather than auditory stimulation alone in training of articulatory errors.
5. training voiced-voiceless distinctions by slowing the speech and concentrating on the correct production of voiceless phonemes; this is critical because it is common for dysarthric cerebral-palsied children to use voiced for voiceless consonants.

Neurologic Symptoms in Articulation

It is important to realize that the production of some sounds is often governed by the degree of oral-motor involvement that the child displays. For instance, as a rule of thumb it is more common for children with dyskinetic dysarthria to have difficulty finding appropriate focal articulation points because of involuntary movement patterns that may be reflected in their oral musculature. Spastics, on the one hand, often have been described as having difficulty in initiating movement and usually display problems in coordination and force in articulation. They often are able to find focal articulation points but have weak and uncoordinated articulatory movement (Platt, Andrews, Young, & Quinn, 1980). Individuals with LMN muscle disorders, on the other hand, often demonstrate muscle weakness but can reach focal articulation points easily while lacking force for articulation. This results in mild to moderate phoneme distortion.

Compensatory Articulation

When a child is unable to produce a speech sound because of apparent neurophysiologic limitations, two options are open to speech-language pathologists. First, they can postpone working on the sounds that appear neurophysiologically impossible until those sounds that can be remediated easily are established. Often with improved articulation skills the child is able to make close approximations of the sound that seemed neurophysiologically impossible at first.

The second option available to speech-language pathologists is to attempt to train a compensatory articulation for normal sounds that are difficult to produce. Often the child will choose a reasonable compensation for the sound without the help of the speech-language pathologist. It is the task of the speech-language pathologist to refine the compensatory sound as much as possible. Sometimes the child chooses a bizarre sound as a compensation. The speech-language pathologist must then redirect the selection of a compensatory sound.

It is important to remember that many dysarthric children will never obtain normality of articulation, and reasonable compensations are often practical and fairly efficient for communication. To take the stance that all compensations should be eliminated is unrealistic for the majority of the childhood dysarthric population. However, for persons with mild speech involvement who may become economically competitive with physically normal peers, striving for near normal or normal articulation may be worth the effort. In other words, projected social demands and expectations in the communication situation may help in setting realistic goals for speech proficiency training.

Frustration in Articulation Therapy

It has been our experience that for most dysarthric children, articulation therapy may be difficult and frustrating. Through the preschool and elementary-school years, it is sometimes wise to give a child a vacation of one to two months after prolonged articulation therapy. This will allow the child to reestablish his resources for what may be an extended total period of time in therapy. It is my belief that articulation therapy deserves vigorous effort on the part of the child and the speech-language pathologist, because much of speech intelligibility lies in articulation skills, particularly tongue function. It has been commonly observed that tongue movements, particularly tongue-tip elevation, are difficult for the neurologically impaired child and often require extensive training for improvement.

Since dysarthric children and their speech-language pathologists often become frustrated at the lack of progress, therapy sometimes is terminated on other grounds than rational ones. This means that during late adolescence or early adulthood dysarthric persons may feel the need to return to a speech-language pathologist to see if more can be done to improve their speech intelligibility. Usually when an individual returns to therapy at an older age, motivation is high and the individual's general maturity will allow him or her to accept further articulation therapy despite moments of frustration.

It is advisable to remember that neurological involvement with severe to moderately severe dysarthria may often demand therapy that is almost a cradle-to-the-grave proposition. In fact, therapy of one sort or another for the rest of their lives may be the destiny of many dysarthric children. We as speech-language pathologists should always be willing to look at a speech case anew and provide encouragement as well as a "refresher course" at any point during the individual's lifetime.

MANAGEMENT OF DEVELOPMENTAL VERBAL DYSPRAXIA

Despite the questionable status of DVD, to provide better therapeutic management, several speech-language pathologists believe that a subgroup of children should be designated as demonstrating DVD. These professionals argue that the therapeutic procedures deemed appropriate for the child with a functional articulation disorder are likely to be inappropriate for a child with suspected DVD. Further, an early diagnosis of DVD may provide a rationale for intensifying therapy, prevent mismanagement, give direction to family counseling, lower expectations for articulation proficiency, and may ultimately lead to the election of an alternate communication device that provides better communication than do oral speech attempts (Jaffe, 1986).

Several management approaches have been reported in the literature, and a given therapy plan may include one or more of these approaches. Some approaches utilize principles employed with acquired apraxia in adults. It is unclear whether the neural mechanisms of adult and child dyspraxia are the same or even similar, but there is a contention among some speech-language pathologists that similar therapy techniques are effective for both groups (Jaffe, 1986).

Diedrich (1982), on the other hand, sees few similarities between adult and child verbal dyspraxics but believes that childhood dyspraxics, dysarthrics, and functional misarticulators are more alike than they are different. The implication is that a similar approach to articulation therapy is probably effective in all three child groups.

The prevailing opinion, however, is that specialized approaches to DVD are usually called for. Many approaches to therapy emphasize specific aspects of traditional articulation therapy but deemphasize other aspects. For example, in their case report of a child suspected of DVD, Love and Fitzgerald (1984) recommend that auditory discrimination drills and rule-based phonologic approaches to articulation training be deemphasized, while imitation of articulatory postures, teaching of phonetic placement, auditory-visual sound stimulation, and motor repetition be stressed. Other approaches reported in the literature, it should be noted, are considered less traditional than is the modified approach to articulation therapy advocated by Love and Fitzgerald.

Some of the several approaches to management of the child with DVD will be discussed later, but before that discussion, it is important to point out that the effectiveness of most DVD treatment programs is essentially unknown (Pannbacker, 1988). There are several problems in the literature of DVD management. Many of the approaches reported have been based on single cases or on a very few children. No reports are available that document the response of a group of DVD children to a given technique. Moreover, many of the reported approaches have not been well-described and could not be replicated satisfactorily. Dyspraxic symptoms reported to have changed because of a certain therapy technique have not been measured objectively nor have appropriate control subjects been employed to demonstrate conclusively that the change in dyspraxic symptoms is a true treatment effect instead of a result of uncontrolled factors. Pannbacker has reviewed the major published reports on management of children with DVD and has summarized the effectiveness in Table 8-1. Study of this table will quickly re-

TABLE 8-1   Therapy Approaches Available for DAS

Type of therapy	Reference	General effectiveness
ACT: Adapted cueing technique	Klick (1985)	Generally untested
Audiometer integration	Chappel (1973)	Untested
Contingencies— Wisconsin test apparatus	Daly et al. (1972)	Preliminary results— efficacious
Hierarchies, movement sequencing, systematic drill	Rosenbek et al. (1974)	Preliminary results— efficacious
Melodic intonation therapy	Doszak et al. (1987) Smith and Engel (1984)	Generally untested
Nonspeech	Harlan (1984)	Generally untested
Prompt System (prompts for restructuring oral muscular phonetic targets)	Chumpelik (1984)	Untested
STP (signed target phoneme)	Shelton and Graves (1985)	Generally untested
Total communication	Jaffe (1984)	Preliminary results— efficacious
Touch-cue system	Bashir et al. (1984)	Untested

Source: Reprinted by permission of the publisher from "Management strategies for developmental apraxia of speech: A review of the literature," by Mary Pannbacker, *Journal of Communication Disorders, 21,* 363-371. Copyright 1988 by Elsevier Science Publishing Co., Inc.

veal that the effectiveness of the management approaches to DVD has not been adequately or scientifically documented.

If there are no proven approaches to therapy for DVD, what is the student of childhood motor speech disability to make of the literature on the management of DVD? First, the speech-language pathologist must study the various approaches and decide which approach or approaches appear to be the most logically and scientifically based and would be the most effective for the child with DVD. Second, after studying Pannbacker's review, the speech-language pathologist may see that several approaches are effective to some degree with the child with DVD, and there is yet no technique of choice.

Traditional Approaches

Many writers, according to Thompson (1988), have advocated a management program that includes using oral-motor and oral-sensory training, developing articulatory postures, training sound sequences, and using speech training associated with rhythm, hand, and/or body movement.

Oral-Motor and Oral-Sensory Training.   Oral exercises have been widely advocated in the treatment of DVD (Haynes, 1985; Yoss & Darley, 1974). Yoss and Darley suggest imitation and mirror work to increase range of motion of muscles, encourage accurate placement of the articulators, and discourage dyspraxic movements of the oral mechanism. Haynes also advocates concentrated drill on movement of the tongue and lips in imitation as well as on command. She asserts that using foods and mouthwash will elicit desired movement patterns. For instance, a patient's tongue tip and right buccal cavity can be swabbed with mouthwash and the patient then can be instructed to move the tongue tip to the designated target site in the right buccal cavity. In addition, the patient can be required to remove food from within the oral cavity with the tongue, and the patient also can be required to use the tongue to remove small bits of food placed on a tongue blade at various distances and angles from the oral cavity. Visual feedback is usually given during these therapy tasks. The goal of the therapy tasks is a heightening of visual sensory awareness of articulatory postures.

Additional sensory awareness techniques used by Haynes (1985) include bombarding the oral-sensory mechanism with multisensory stimuli. In particular, tactile stimulation is stressed because of presumed facilitation of the pyramidal tract, which executes skilled and planned movements for articulation. Additional stimulating techniques include using textures, such as cotton or sandpaper applied to the patient's upper lip, tongue, palate, and buccal area. Deep pressure and resistance techniques are also employed to facilitate oral awareness. However, as pointed out earlier, the role of oral-sensory function in the speech mechanism is at best equivocal, and it is difficult to assess whether these techniques of oral awareness facilitation are really beneficial. Research on the effectiveness of oral-sensory facilitation in a DVD management program is urgently needed.

Developing Articulatory Postures.   Although the development of articulatory postures is highlighted in some treatment programs, Rosenbek, Hansen, Baughman, and Lemme (1974) and Jaffe (1986) are opposed to the practice because the child with DVD often finds it extremely difficult to imitate the articulatory postures of the speech-language pathologist. However, Haynes (1985), Blakeley (1983), and Logue (1978) all employ in their total programs some aspect of the development of articulatory gestures. For instance, to develop vowel posture, Blakeley suggests observing your own mouth in a mirror and then placing manually the child's tongue and lips into a like posture and position, asking the child to "make a noise" for training vowel production (p. 32). Blakeley believes that even during neutral phonation the child's tongue and lips can be shaped into different vowels.

Training Sound Sequences.   The inability to sequence sounds is usually described as a critical, if not a defining, feature of DVD. Therapy therefore is often directed toward this aspect of the disorder (Haynes, 1985; Rosenbek et al., 1974; Yoss & Darley, 1974). Usually, meaningful stimuli are employed beginning with the production of visible consonants in CV, VC, and CVC sequences and then proceeding to words and phrases. Haynes (1985), for one, has advocated the use of the intrusive schwa when DVD children have difficulty with complex sound clusters. Research, however, is unavailable to determine how effective sound sequencing training with an intrusive schwa really is.

Speech Training Associated with Rhythm, Hand, and/or Body Movement.
Haynes (1985) has indicated that nonspeech behaviors, such as foot tapping or finger tapping, are helpful in the treatment of DVD. It is believed that these activities tend to highlight sequence and changes in the placement of the articulators. With the same goal in mind, many of the less traditional approaches described for treatment of DVD incorporate manual or rhythmic movement as one aspect of a total therapy plan.

Other Approaches

Several other approaches have been reported for managing DVD, but as Pannbacker (1988) has pointed out, they all remain somewhat suspect until more data becomes available confirming their efficacy for DVD management. Some of these approaches are reviewed briefly in the following paragraphs.

Klick (1985) has used adapted cueing techniques (ACT) from the manual alphabet for the deaf to enhance oral stimuli and elicit more correct articulations. Bashir, Grahamjones, and Bostwick (1984) have developed a tactile cueing method called the "touch-cue method." Shelton and Graves (1985) have used hand shapes from the American Manual Alphabet for Signed Target Phonemes to work with a 5-year-old boy. Harlan (1984) has reported the use of concurrent nonspeech, signed English, and oral-motor treatment for a 3-year-old dyspraxic, arguing that early intervention and alternate communication techniques were justified by the child's success.

Chumpelik (1984) has reported the use of a system that included tactile stimulation and phonetic placement procedures. The system, called

PROMPTS (Prompts for Restructuring Oral Muscular Phonetic Targets), was considered successful by the author. Daly, Cantrill, Cantrill, and Aman (1972) have employed the *Wisconsin Test Apparatus* to provide feedback for correct responses. A severely apraxic child was treated for six months, and positive changes were reported.

Melodic Intonation Therapy (MIT), a singing technique used first with adult aphasics, was employed by Dozak, McNeil, and Jaccosek (1981) with an apraxic child. Helfrich-Miller (1984) has combined MIT and total communication and reported gains in two children. Last, a palatal lift prosthesis has recently been used to manage hypernasality in a suspected DVD case (Hall, Hardy, & LaVelle, 1990).

DVD Research.   Limited research is available on therapy techniques for dyspraxic individuals. Therefore, it is probably appropriate to end this chapter by giving a summary of one of the few research studies on the management of individuals with suspected DVD. More important is the fact that the design for study may point the way toward the type of scientific research that is desperately needed in the future to solve the controversy surrounding DVD therapy effectiveness.

Young and Thompson (1987) and Thompson (1988) have described a controlled study on one aspect of the management of suspected DVD. The subjects of the research were two adults, both of whom had been diagnosed in their youth as DVD children. This study employed a multiple baseline design for single subjects. The two subjects were trained to produce initial word fricatives plus a liquid and fricative and stop clusters as well as ambisyllabic or abutting consonants in bisyllabic words. These sounds and sound clusters have often been reported to be particularly difficult for DVD children.

In this research, target words were trained with rebus-cued training procedures. In these techniques, colored pictures of target nouns were trained with backward chaining. For instance, a picture of the noun *magnet* and a picture of the rebus *net* were presented with the rebus first and the whole word next. By imitating through a succession of steps, subjects learned to say the target words without the rebus. Results indicated that training was effective for both subjects in enhancing the production of abutting consonants in bisyllabic words and in initial consonants. Generalization to untrained sounds occurred, although one subject showed greater generalization than the other. Generalization to spontaneous speech was not studied.

In a sense, this study provides a model for future attempts to validate DVD therapy procedures. In particular, single-subject multiple-baseline studies allow the investigator to deal with the problem of a limited number of subjects, a hallmark of the population who may be truly dyspraxic. The multiple-baseline design employing two subjects rather than one, of course, allows much greater control and ability to generalize than does the usual controlled case study report of the effectiveness of a treatment program in DVD. Clearly, more single-subject studies of therapy, such as this one, are needed to resolve the puzzle of DVD management.

Since the first edition of this book, a seminar entitled "Dynamic Remediation Strategies for Children with Developmental Verbal Dyspraxia," by Shelly L. Velleman and Kristine E. Strand (1998), has been distributed by the American Speech-Language-Hearing Association. The seminar advocates a phonotaxic perspective and provides a suggested treatment program that aims at increasing early grammatical skills in children with DVD. Academic language patterns of children with DVD are presented. Current literary concepts are discussed to provide a basis for the reading and writing deficits found in children with DVD. The seminar is videotaped and accompanied by a 90-page manual that includes training materials and a self-study program for continuing education credit with the American Speech-Language-Hearing Association education program. The videotaped seminar and the accompanying training manual are an impressive contribution to the clinical literature on DVD that has been written since 1992.

SUMMARY

The majority of this chapter describes a speech subsystems approach to therapy planning and management of childhood dysarthria. It assumes that careful analysis of the functions and dysfunctions of each speech subsystem in the neurologically impaired child will provide information to determine how and where to intervene to improve speech performance. A subsystems analysis is usually initiated only after the child has completed a program of prespeech feeding to increase and improve the movement patterns of the oropharyngeal muscles. An accompanying program of stimulating and reinforcing vocal play is integrated with the prespeech feeding program (see Chapter 7).

When the child begins formal speech training, generally the first area to be considered is management of respiratory dysfunction. An initial step is to provide an appropriate positioning and physical support for speaking. Development of head balance, normal neck extension, continuing head support, and appropriate shoulder and trunk alignment with a slightly flexed sitting posture all help to enhance development of good breath support for speech production.

Attempting to increase physiologic support for speech is useful, but it must be realized that the degree of motor involvement of the respiratory muscles may impose limitations on the ultimate speech breathing performance. Despite the degree of involvement, the child must be taught to talk within the physiological limits of the respiratory system. Training to increase the capacity for air intake, training for prolonged vowel production, and teaching the child to speak at relatively high lung volumes are valuable activities in this regard. Generally, sustained blowing activities are contraindicated since control for blowing and speech production is dissimilar. However, the training of conscious speech phrasing within the limits of tidal air flow generally increases overall intelligibility of speech. Improved speech phrasing and use of a slower rate may be enhanced by using a pacing board.

Both hypo- and hyperfunctional vocal symptoms are present in childhood dysarthria. Some experts suggest a trial of therapy but are generally pessimistic about achieving improvement in children with severe vocal disturbances. Voice management in adolescents with cerebral palsy is sometimes effective because early speech therapy often concentrates heavily on articulation improvement, not voice therapy. Traditional techniques involving recognition of vocal deviations, auditory discrimination, and audio- or videotape monitoring of vocal production are often surprisingly effective.

Reduced tonus in laryngeal muscles in flaccid dysarthrias may not be reversible by using traditional "pushing" exercises; portable voice amplifiers may be considered as augmentative aids in such cases. Instruments such as *Visipitch* (Kay Elemetrics) are often helpful in modifying pitch disturbances. Use of simple diagrams to train rising and falling pitch contours is also useful in developing speech naturalness. Identification of target linguistic stress improves prosodic disturbances.

Velopharyngeal dysfunction has been identified as a common problem in childhood dysarthria, and particular attention has been paid to the problem in the cerebral-palsied. Of the three basic approaches to the problem—palatal exercise, palatal lift prosthesis, and palatal surgery—the palatal lift prosthesis appears to be the most effective in a dysarthria characterized by severe hypernasality and poor oral pharyngeal control. If the palatal lift cannot be fitted, the next option usually is pharyngeal flap surgery.

Articulation therapy, particularly correcting phonetic placement errors, has always had high priority in speech habilitation programs. Whether articulation training should be preceded by a regime of oral resistance exercises is debatable, but intensive articulation training is beneficial with or without muscle training in most childhood dysarthrias. Resistance exercises are probably beneficial in selected cases of muscle weakness. Phonologic process testing and management planning appear to be useful in articulation therapy although limited evidence of their use is available in childhood dysarthria cases. Phonemes requiring greater motor complexity are frequently in error in dysarthria and point up the overriding factor of neurologic involvement in articulation production. Compensatory articulations must be taught when neurologic involvement is severe. Intensive articulation therapy often results in frustration for the child, and provisions must be made to relieve the frustration, usually through periodic therapeutic vacations, if articulation habilitation is to be successful. If unintelligibility remains, augmentative communication technology may be needed.

Management of DVD is controversial. Many speech-language pathologists advocate specialized approaches to this uncommon articulation disorder, which is often resistant to therapy. Traditional approaches in DVD management emphasize imitation of articulatory postures and teaching of phonetic placements; these approaches deemphasize auditory discrimination and rule-based phonologic treatment. Oral-sensory stimulation and training are emphasized along with the teaching of sound sequencing. Speech training is associated with rhythmic patterns of hand and body movements in traditional approaches.

A series of reports have appeared that emphasize new techniques or a combination of techniques, such as various types of cueing, use of the manual alphabet, signed English, alternate communication, melodic intonation, total communication, and palatal lift prosthesis. Although each anecdotal report has claimed varying degrees of success with individual cases of suspected DVD and several appear promising, it is important to replicate the success reported with other DVD cases to establish the validity of specific therapeutic techniques. It is regrettable that since the first edition of this book in 1992 no replication research studies have appeared in the literature to try to verify the therapeutic techniques presented in the more promising clinical studies used in the treatment of children suspected of DVD.

SUGGESTED READING

Netsell, R., Lotz, W. K., & Barlow, S. M. (1989). A speech physiology examination for individuals with dysarthria. In K. M. Yorkston & D. R. Beukelman (Eds.), *Recent advances in clinical dysarthria* (pp. 3–37). Boston: Little, Brown.

This chapter illustrates a laboratory approach to the analysis of speech subsystem dysfunction. This technique is applicable to both child and adult. Implications for therapy are apparent.

Thompson, C. K. (1988). Articulation disorders in the child with neurogenic pathology. In N. J. Lass, L. V. McReynolds, J. L. Northern, and D. E. Yoder (Eds.), *Handbook of speech-language pathology and audiology* (pp. 548–591). Toronto: B. C. Decker.

Thompson provides an up-to-date management approach for childhood dysarthria based on a subsystems concept of therapy, and she reviews the current status of the management of DVD.

REFERENCES

Aronson, A. (1985). *Clinical voice disorders* (2nd ed.). New York: Thieme-Stratton.
Barlow, S. M. (1989). A high-speed data acquisition system for clinical speech physiology. In K. M. Yorkston & D. R. Beukelman (Eds.), *Recent advances in clinical dysarthria* (pp. 39–52). Boston: Little, Brown.

Barlow, S., & Farley, G. R. (1989). Neurophysiology of speech. In D. P. Kuehn, M. L. Lemme, & J. M. Baumgartner (Eds.), *Neural bases of speech, hearing and language* (pp. 146–200). Boston: Little, Brown.

Bashir, A. S., Grahamjones, F., & Bostwick, R.Y. (1984). A touch-cue method of therapy for developmental apraxia of speech. *Seminars in Speech and Language, 5,* 127–137.

Blakeley, R. W. (1983). Treatment of developmental apraxia of speech. In W. H. Perkins (Ed.), *Dysarthria and apraxia* (pp. 25–33). New York: Thieme-Stratton.

Canter, G. (1965). Speech characteristics of patients with Parkinson's disease: II. Physiologic support for speech. *Journal of Speech and Hearing Disorders, 30,* 217–224.

Chumpelik, D. (1984). The prompt system of therapy: Theoretical framework and applications for developmental apraxia of speech. *Seminars in Speech and Language, 5,* 139–155.

Cole, R. M. (1971). Direct muscle training for the improvement of velopharyngeal function. In W. C. Grabb, S. W. Rosenstein, & K. R. Bzoch (Eds.), *Cleft lip and palate* (pp. 328–340). Boston: Little, Brown.

Crary, M. A., & Comeau, S. (1981). Phonologically based assessment and intervention in spastic cerebral palsy: A case analysis. *South African Journal of Communication Disorders, 28,* 29–37.

Daly, D. A., Cantrill, R. P., Cantrill, M. L., & Aman, L. A. (1972). Structuring speech therapy contingencies with an oral apraxic child. *Journal of Speech and Hearing Disorders, 37,* 22–32.

Darley, F. L., Aronson, A. E., & Brown, J. R. (1975). *Motor speech disorders.* Philadelphia: W. B. Saunders.

Diedrich, W. (1982). Toward an understanding of communication disorders. In N. Lass, L. McReynolds, J. Northern, & D. Yoder (Eds.), *Speech, language, hearing. Volume II: Pathologies of speech and language.* Philadelphia: W. B. Saunders.

Dozak, A., McNeil, M., & Jaccosek, E. (1981). *Efficacy of melodic intonation therapy with developmental apraxia of speech.* Paper presented at the annual convention of the American Speech-Language-Hearing Association, Los Angeles.

Fisher, H. B., & Logemann, J. A. (1971). *The Fisher-Logemann Test of Articulation Competence.* Boston: Houghton Mifflin.

Froeschels, E. (1952). *Dysarthric speech.* Magnolia, MA: Expression.

Froeschels, E., Kastein, S., & Weiss, D. A. (1955). A method of therapy for paralytic conditions of the mechanisms of phonation, respiration, and glutination. *Journal of Speech and Hearing Disorders, 20,* 356–370.

Hall, P. K., Hardy, J. C., & LaVelle, W. E. (1990). A child with signs of developmental apraxia of speech with whom a palatal lift prosthesis was used to manage palatal dysfunction. *Journal of Speech and Hearing Disorders, 55,* 454–460.

Hardy, J. C. (1964). Lung function of athetoid and spastic quadriplegic children. *Developmental Medicine and Child Neurology, 6,* 378–388.

Hardy, J. C. (1983). *Cerebral palsy.* Englewood Cliffs, NJ: Prentice Hall.

Hardy, J. C., & Edmonds, T. D. (1968). Electronic integrator for measurement of partitions of the lung volume. *Journal of Speech and Hearing Research, 11,* 777–786.

Hardy, J. C., Rembolt, R., Spriesterbach, D., & Jaypathy, B. (1961). Surgical management of palatal paresis and speech problems in cerebral palsy: A preliminary report. *Journal of Speech and Hearing Disorders, 26,* 320–325.

Harlan, N. T. (1984). Treatment approaches for a young child evidencing developmental verbal apraxia. *Australian Journal of Human Communication Disorders, 12,* 121–127.

Haynes, S. (1985). Developmental apraxia of speech: Symptoms and treatment. In D. F. Johns (Ed.), *Clinical management of neurogenic communication disorders* (2nd ed., pp. 259–266). Boston: Little, Brown.

Helfrich-Miller, K. (1984). Melodic intonation therapy with developmentally apraxic children. *Seminars in Speech and Language, 5,* 119–126.

Helm, N. A. (1979). Management of palilalia with a pacing board. *Journal of Speech and Hearing Disorders, 44,* 350–353.

Hixon, T., Hawley, J., & Wilson, J. (1982). An around-the-house device for the clinical determination of respiratory driving pressure: A note on making simple even simpler. *Journal of Speech and Hearing Disorders, 47,* 413.

Jaffe, M. B. (1986). Neurologic impairment of speech production: Assessment and treatment. In A. Holland & J. M. Costello (Eds.), *Handbook of speech and language disorders* (pp. 157–186). San Diego: College Hill Press.

Klick, S. (1985). Adapted cueing technique for use in treatment of dyspraxia. *Language, Speech, and Hearing Services in Schools, 16,* 256–259.

LaVelle, W. E., & Hardy, J. C. (1979). Palatal lift prosthesis for the treatment of palatopharyngeal incompetence. *Journal of Prosthetic Dentistry, 42,* 308–315.

Logue, R. D. (1978). Disorders of motor-speech planning in children: Evaluation and treatment. *Communication disorders: An audio-journal for continuing education, 3.* New York: Grune & Stratton.

Lotz, W. K., & Netsell, R. (1989). Velopharyngeal management for a child with dysarthria and cerebral palsy. In K. M. Yorkston & D. R. Beukelman (Eds.), *Recent advances in clinical dysarthria* (pp. 139–143). Boston: Little, Brown.

Love, R. J., & Fitzgerald, M. (1984). Is the diagnosis of developmental apraxia of speech valid? *Australian Journal of Human Communication Disorders, 12,* 170–178.

McDonald, E. T., & Chance, B., Jr. (1964). *Cerebral palsy.* Englewood Cliffs, NJ: Prentice Hall.

McWilliams, B. J., Morris, H. L., & Shelton, R. (1990). *Cleft palate speech* (2nd ed.). Ontario: B. C. Decker.

Musselwhite, C. R., & St. Louis, K. W. (1988). *Communication programming for persons with severe handicaps: Vocal and augmentative strategies* (2nd ed.). Boston: Little, Brown.

Netsell, R. (1969). Evaluation of velopharyngeal function in dysarthria. *Journal of Speech & Hearing Disorders, 34,* 113–122.

Netsell, R., & Daniel, B. (1979). Dysarthria in adults: Physiologic approach to rehabilitation. *Archives of Physical Medicine & Rehabilitation, 60,* 502–508.

Netsell, R., Lotz, W. K., & Barlow, S. M. (1989). A speech physiology examination for individuals with dysarthria. In K. M. Yorkston & D. R. Beukelman (Eds.), *Recent advances in clinical dysarthria* (pp. 3–37). Boston: Little, Brown.

Pannbacker, M. (1988). Management strategies for developmental apraxia of speech: A review of the literature. *Journal of Communication Disorders, 21,* 367–371.

Platt, L., Andrews, G., Young, M., & Quinn, P. (1980). Dysarthria of adult cerebral palsy: II. Phonemic analysis of articulatory errors. *Journal of Speech and Hearing Research, 23,* 41–55.

Porter, P. B., Wurth, B., & Stowers, S. (1988). Seating and positioning for communication. In D. E. Yoder & R. D. Kent (Eds.), *Decision making in speech-language pathology*. Toronto: B. C. Decker.

Putnam, A., & Hixon, T. J. (1984). Respiratory kinematics in speakers with motor neuron disease. In M. McNeil, J. Rosenbek, & A. Aronson (Eds.), *The dysarthrias*. San Diego, CA: College Hill Press.

Rosenbek, J., Hansen, R., Baughman, C. H., & Lemme, M. (1974). Treatment of developmental apraxia of speech: A case study. *Language, Speech, and Hearing Services in Schools, 5,* 13–22.

Rosenbek, J. C., & LaPointe, L. L. (1985). The dysarthrias: Description, diagnosis and treatment. In D. E. Johns (Ed.), *Clinical management of neurogenic communicative disorders* (2nd ed., pp. 97–152). Boston: Little, Brown.

Ruscello, D. (1982). A selected review of palatal training procedures. *Cleft Palate Journal, 19,* 181–194.

Salomonson, J., Kawamoto, H., & Wilson, L. (1988). Velopharyngeal incompetence as the presenting symptom of myotonic dystrophy. *Cleft Palate Journal, 25,* 296–300.

Shelton, M., & Graves, M. (1985). Use of visual techniques in therapy for developmental apraxia of speech. *Language, Speech, and Hearing Services in Schools, 16,* 129–131.

Strand, K. E., & Velleman, S. L. (1998). Seminar: Dynamic remediation strategies for children with developmental verbal dyspraxia. Pittsburgh, PA: Rehab Training Network and the American Speech-Language-Hearing Association.

Thompson, C. K. (1988). Articulation disorders in the child with neurogenic pathology. In N. J. Lass, L. V. McReynolds, J. L. Northern, & D. E. Yoder (Eds.), *Handbook of speech-language pathology and audiology* (pp. 548–591). Toronto: B. C. Decker.

Westlake, H., & Rutherford, D. (1961). *Speech therapy for the cerebral palsied*. Chicago: National Society for Crippled Children and Adults.

Yorkston, K. M., Beukelman, D. R., & Bell, K. R. (1986). *Clinical management of dysarthric speakers*. Boston: Little, Brown.

Yoss, K. A., & Darley, F. L. (1974). Therapy in developmental apraxia of speech. *Language, Speech, and Hearing Services in Schools, 5,* 23–31.

Young, E. C., & Thompson, C. K. (1987). An experimental analysis of treatment effects on consonant clusters and ambisyllabic consonants in two adults with developmental phonological problems. *Journal of Communication Disorders, 20,* 137–149.

Index